T0157753

Heart to Heart

12 People Discover Better Lives after Their Heart Attacks

C. BRUCE JOHNSON

iUniverse, Inc.
New York   Bloomington

Copyright © 2009 by C. Bruce Johnson

All rights reserved. No part of this book may be used or reproduced by any means, graphic, electronic, or mechanical, including photocopying, recording, taping or by any information storage retrieval system without the written permission of the publisher except in the case of brief quotations embodied in critical articles and reviews.

The information, ideas, and suggestions in this book are not intended as a substitute for professional medical advice. Before following any suggestions contained in this book, you should consult your personal physician. Neither the author nor the publisher shall be liable or responsible for any loss or damage allegedly arising as a consequence of your use or application of any information or suggestions in this book.

iUniverse books may be ordered through booksellers or by contacting:

iUniverse
1663 Liberty Drive
Bloomington, IN 47403
www.iuniverse.com
1-800-Authors (1-800-288-4677)

Because of the dynamic nature of the Internet, any Web addresses or links contained in this book may have changed since publication and may no longer be valid. The views expressed in this work are solely those of the author and do not necessarily reflect the views of the publisher, and the publisher hereby disclaims any responsibility for them.

ISBN: 978-1-4401-7075-1 (sc)
ISBN: 978-1-4401-7076-8 (ebook)
ISBN: 978-1-4401-7074-4 (dj)

Printed in the United States of America

iUniverse rev. date: 10/30/2009

Contents

Foreword..vii

Acknowledgments xi

Introduction xv

Chapter 1: My Story..1

Chapter 2: Steve Sobelman..27

Chapter 3: Erin Peiffer 46

Chapter 4: Hurst Bousegard...63

Chapter 5: Anita Fox..84

Chapter 6: Evan Kushner...99

Chapter 7: The Reverend James Love.......................................112

Chapter 8: Mary Maguire 129

Chapter 9: Morris Ginsberg..143

Chapter 10: Neal Gregory..162

Chapter 11: Barbara Robinson...173

Chapter 12: Larry Harris 186

Conclusion 199

American Heart Association Recommended Links 201

Foreword

Since the beginning of time, the heart has been the subject of poets and philosophers. But this marvelous organ, which contracts over a trillion times—flawlessly in most individuals—can become a traitor, ending life in an instant or leaving its victim's health seriously compromised.

Individual responses to heart attacks are varied. For many reasons, half of the victims don't survive. Those who do are changed forever. Many patients respond positively with changes in lifestyles, risk-factor modification, diets, and adherence to medications. Others cannot manage those changes, and their heart disease defeats them. It is the duty of all of us in the health-care field to help patients respond in a positive manner. That way our compliant patients become healthier and serve as role models to others to help them through this difficult period.

Veteran broadcast journalist Bruce Johnson is a heart-attack survivor, and he wants to get the word out on how to take back one's life after being hit with this lightning bolt. In *Heart to Heart*, he tells not only his own story, sixteen years in the making, but he also relates the stories of eleven other courageous people, men and women, young and not so young, who looked death in the face and lived to tell about it.

In the early 1960s, the treatment for a heart attack consisted of admission to a general medical floor, morphine for pain, and oxygen delivered through a nasal cannula; subsequently, patients were confined to bed for weeks or months. Blood thinners were used only to militate against blood clots forming in the legs because of inactivity. The mortality rate of such patients was 25 percent after they reached the hospital. Over the next decade, it was learned that patients died because of irregularities of the heart rhythm that could be corrected. Special coronary-care units isolated these patients, continuous electrocardiogram monitoring was instituted, and nurses were empowered to treat potentially fatal arrhythmias with cardioversion shocks. These protocols were very effective and reduced the hospital mortality of heart-attack victims by half. A decade later, it became clear that heart attacks, which would subsequently be referred to as acute myocardial infarctions, were caused by blood clots spontaneously occurring in the coronary arteries (a condition known as coronary thrombosis). The possibility of dissolving these clots with intravenous medications known as thrombolytics, or "clot busters," was explored, and the clinical trials were positive, with the mortality of patients being reduced. Percutaneous coronary intervention—more commonly known as angioplasty—in which coronary obstructions are dilated with a balloon, was evolving as a useful technique in stable patients with coronary blockages and was found to be effective in treating these thrombotic coronary obstructions. Almost two decades later, the issue is not whether to perform angioplasty, but how quickly we can do it. The standard of care is to perform these procedures less than 90 minutes from the onset of symptoms.

This is a challenge even during the regular workday, with personnel available for such emergencies. But because most heart attacks occur in the early morning hours, when cardiac-catheterization laboratory staffs are not usually in hospitals, it has been even harder to meet this goal. Thousands of hospitals are responding to this challenge, however, and are committing the resources to achieve this end. The evolution of the field of cardiac care has been rapid and has produced the desired result: a reduced mortality rate among heart-attack victims.

Bruce Johnson received the thrombolytic clot-busting drugs and later had an angioplasty. Today, nearly twenty years later, because hospitals have committed more resources, and physicians have heeded the call, a blocked coronary artery can be more predictably opened, in most patients, with a stent in less than two hours, 24/7. These techniques and adjunctive medications have reduced the hospital mortality of heart-attack victims from 25 percent in the 1960s to about 5 percent now.

Because there are over one million heart attacks in the U.S. each year, this means many more lives are being saved. Armed with this encouraging information, health-care providers can be far more persuasive with their patients when discussing risk-factor modifications and prescribed drugs that have proven successful in helping control blood pressure, heart rates, and cholesterol levels. The damper on this positive news is the undeniable increase in body weight among Americans in the at-risk population. Predictably, this has led to an increase in the incidence of diabetes and the terrible effect that has on vascular disease. Cigarette smoking remains far too prevalent and is one of the more difficult risk factors to control. Although challenges remain, we have made much progress with heart disease, which nevertheless remains our most prevalent life-threatening problem.

Bruce Johnson survived his initial heart attack. He made important changes in his lifestyle. He has lived to share not only his own valuable story but those of others.

Following heart attacks, all patients and all families of patients need guidance. The stories in *Heart to Heart* serve to emphasize the benefits of maintaining a positive response, allowing others to help with your recovery, taking charge of one's destiny, and being a beneficiary of four decades of science and technology.

Kenneth Kent, MD
Washington Hospital Center

Acknowledgments

This book would still be just an important thought forever locked in my mind had I not been able to find the eleven other people whose stories are told in these pages.

I will forever be grateful to Steve Sobelman, Mary Maguire, Larry Harris, Barbara Robinson, Anita Fox, Hurst Bousegard, Morris Ginsburg, the Reverend James Love, Evan Kushner, Neal Gregory, and Erin Peiffer. I thank them for their time, their honest sharing, and their patience with this project. They could have remained anonymous but chose to share their stories, their setbacks, and their successes in hopes of helping others. You will come to know them—and maybe even love them—as I do. They are the true heroes in *Heart to Heart*.

I want to thank Jonathan Hemmerdinger, my hard-working research and writing assistant. Jon is a graduate student in journalism at Georgetown University. He came highly recommended by a friend and colleague, Barbara Feinman Todd, associate dean at Georgetown who has collaborated with Bob Woodward and Hillary Clinton on book projects.

Christina Weaver came on board early and volunteered to help with research, interviews, and organizing my scattered thoughts.

Lynn Adrine also helped me stay focused. Over dinner she reminded me to do what I do best, "just report and tell their stories."

The doctors, nurses, and communications staff at the Washington Hospital Center were simply incredible at helping recall my own story and making sure my medical information was on the mark.

My personal cardiologist, Dr. Joseph Robinson, gets special thanks here. JR has become a great friend and sounding board on everything. His staff often complains that the laugher that comes out of his office during my visits makes it difficult to carry on phone conversations with other inquiring patients.

The late Dr. Hector Collison helped save my life. Enough said!

I will never be able to give the thanks he deserves to Dr. Kenneth Kent, noted cardiologist and author of more than two hundred published articles, for his contributions and written introduction. My wife and I cried one night after reading one of his e-mails in which he described *Heart to Heart* as a "fabulous" and needed project.

The American Heart Association has been a major inspiration over the years.

Special thanks go to Darcy Alison Spitz, senior communications manager for the AHA in New York. Darcy provided the important links, recommended by the AHA staff that can be found at the end of my book.

Special thanks also go out to Mended Hearts, the AHA's national support group for heart patients and their families.

I needed several editors for this project, including Laura Strachan, my literary agent for another book project. Laura's critiques led to many late nights and weekend writing sessions when my body begged for some time off.

Ron Silverman provided the final editing, asking the tough questions necessary to make sure that what ended up on paper was what I was actually attempting to convey. Thanks, Ron.

The writing for this book really began on July 2, 1992. I want to thank my cameraman, Michael Fox, who got me to the fire station that day; and the paramedics who rushed me to Greater Southeast Community Hospital, which today has been transformed into the first-rate United Medical Center, with some of the same people who worked in the emergency room the afternoon I arrived in cardiac arrest.

My family has been steadfast all along. My wife and best friend, Lori Smith Johnson, believed in this project from the start and would often ask, "How is the book coming?" Translation: "You're going to finish this, right?"

My daughter and son, Kurshanna and Brandon, were encouraging from the beginning and offered their own private thoughts in this book about how my ordeal affected them. Madge Johnson, my former wife, has been equally supportive and also contributed to *Heart to Heart*. Thanks Madge.

Thanks Carolyn, Shawn, Miles, Stephanie, Anthony, and Braydon.

Finally, I want to thank my mother, Mary Johnson Marbry, who passed away before I could get started on *Heart to Heart*. After my heart attack, she would remind me of how blessed I had been. I always agreed, and then we would both ponder, not so much about why I was spared while others suffer the same massive coronary and die, but about what I should do with the rest of this life. I love you Mom. Miss you.

Introduction

I was on vacation in my favorite spot in Lewes, Delaware, near the Atlantic Ocean, when Michael Jackson, the King of Pop, was rushed to a hospital in cardiac arrest.

My first thoughts were probably no different from everybody else's that day: shock and disbelief. Oh, no, he's too young. It's way too soon for Michael to go, and certainly not because of a heart attack;

Then I remembered my own medical history and how I had a sudden heart attack while on the job as a hard-charging TV reporter. Michael Jackson, the world's greatest entertainer, the singer who gave us "Thriller" and "Billy Jean," the inventor of the moonwalk, was actually closer to my age than my children's. He was nearly fifty-one years old, a late baby boomer. I was only forty-two at the time of my heart attack. My thoughts went from *How could Michael die of a heart attack?* to *Why not Michael?*

It really doesn't matter what sparked the sudden myocardial infarction (MI), the medical term for a heart attack. This is an equal opportunity killer, striking down men, women, young, old, rich, poor, famous, and people who aren't known outside their families and workplaces.

Dead is dead, and by most accounts Michael Jackson and others who died of heart attacks might have been spared had they made a few important lifestyle changes. That's what my doctor and the country's other cardiologists are begging for today.

Cardiovascular disease is the leading cause of death in this country and many other industrialized nations. TV pitchman Billy Mays died in his sleep at age fifty. An autopsy revealed he had been suffering from heart disease.

San Francisco 49ers lineman Thomas Herrion was only twenty-three when he collapsed and died following a preseason game.

NBC-TV moderator Tim Russert, at fifty-eight, was struck by a heart attack on the job on a Friday the 13th in 2008 while preparing for another edition of "Meet the Press."

And then there was twenty-four-year-old Army Sergeant Glen Allison, who died of a heart attack less than a week after arriving to fight in Iraq. His mother, back in Pittsville, Pennsylvania, said he had been in perfect shape.

Half of all heart-attack victims are women, but for some reason, fewer women than men survive heart attacks. Breast cancer gets most of the public's attention, but the fact is that six times as many women will die this year of cardiovascular disease as will die of breast cancer.

While much has been written about the medical side of this disease, little has been written about the human side. That's the purpose—the motivation—behind my book. We're hoping to save a lot of lives with *Heart to Heart*.

In *Heart to Heart*, Evan Kushner, a young Boston attorney, learns to cope with the fear of an early death after suffering a heart attack at age thirty-three.

Rev. James Love, a Washington-area minister, suffers a heart attack in the pulpit, then introduces his entire church to a new, heart-healthy way of life.

Erin Peiffer, of suburban Baltimore, found new meaning in life after losing her six-figure income, corporate career, and health insurance to heart disease.

You'll meet a Wall Street trader who said goodbye to a life of excess, a New Orleans oil-rigger who learns to live without sex, and a marathon runner who finds in his family the strength to cope.

In *Heart to Heart*, I begin with my own story, which I must admit has been difficult to put down on paper. There are some admissions of rather reckless behavior and deep family secrets that make for a sometimes painful yet edge-of-your-seat story. My heart attack enabled me to turn the page to an entirely new way of living.

For my book, I interviewed dozens of people to find a diverse group of heart-attack survivors who represented a cross section of America. I found them, and, in some cases, they heard about my project and found me. In one case, I had put an appeal on my Facebook page for heart-attack survivors to contact me. A Facebook friend whom I had never met personally put me in touch with Evan Kushner. He flew to Washington, and we instantly became a temporary support group of two recovering heart-attack patients.

Several cardiologists who know the power of one patient talking to another put me in touch with other people profiled in *Heart to Heart*. Those doctors told me this book should not wait to be published. Heart disease can be arrested, they insisted.

The people profiled here suffered from heart attacks and cardiovascular disease, and they agreed to share their stories in hopes that readers and their loved ones won't have to go through the same trials and tribulations. Jobs and homes were lost. Self-worth was often tested. In some instances, family and friends disappeared. Marriages and relationships ended. Lives had to be rebuilt along with health.

Most of these people came to epitomize the human spirit and were able to help this reporter tell their stories in ways that will empower others to make better health choices before a heart attack—or to fight back and become their own best advocate should an MI put them or a family member temporarily on the sidelines.

In *Heart to Heart* you will learn how a heart attack can change your life, but you will also learn where to find strength to get on with the *rest* of your life.

I hope everyone touched by heart disease—survivors, families, doctors—will read and share this book. I've been a broadcast journalist for many years. Helping get the word out about beating heart attacks is no doubt my biggest assignment to date.

Chapter 1:   My Story

The pain was intense and unrelenting, and I immediately thought someone had shot me. My hands moved to my chest to put pressure on a hemorrhage that wasn't there. No blood. No hole in my starched, white dress shirt. I tore open the top buttons and pulled at the tie around my neck to get more air. The pain was somewhere deep in my chest, where I couldn't get to it.

My good friend and cameraman, Mike Fox, was driving.

"Damn, turn off the air."

I thought the contrast of the air conditioning in the car with Washington's summer heat and humidity might be causing the problem. Maybe it was just indigestion from the greasy burger I devoured at yet another lunch on the run. The pain pressed on, like a vise tightening my chest.

"Stop the car. Maybe I can walk it off." The news car pulled over to the curb on Stanton Road in Southeast. I knew the area well. I had done stories inside the elementary school that stood in the middle of the block. Shortly after I moved to D.C. from my first TV job in Cincinnati, I assigned myself to the rough Stanton Dwellings Public Housing project with another cameraman and friend, Mike Murphy. We documented the daily twists and turns in the lives of Stanton Dwellings resident Barbara Price and her children.

Walking a few steps didn't ease the pain in my chest. It hadn't moved to my arm or anywhere else. I was worried, but not panicked. After all, I was only forty-two, in good shape, a tough street reporter in a tough town that critics like to refer to as "Murder Capital" of the country. I often took my camera crews into neighborhoods where some cops wouldn't dare go alone.

"Mike, get me to a hospital," I gasped. "Let's go to GW."

George Washington University Hospital is where President Ronald Reagan was taken when John Hinckley shot him in 1981, and it was on the way back to Channel 9. I was thinking, *GW saved the president. It can save me too.* They could check me out, and I could still make it to the station and get my story written and edited for the 6 p.m. news. Truth was, I didn't want to go to the neighborhood health-care facility, Greater Southeast Community Hospital. I had covered stories about horrible conditions there: uninsured patients, inadequate staff. It was a hospital with multimillion-dollar deficits that was unable to keep its accreditation. I feel bad saying it now, but honestly, if this turned out to be serious, I didn't want them cutting me up at Greater Southeast.

The pain wouldn't let up. Eventually I decided it was time to panic and began to worry that I wasn't going to make it across the Anacostia River through downtown to GW.

Mike had sensed something wasn't right with me all day long. He said I had been complaining most of the day—"bitchin" is the word he used. He said I seemed preoccupied.

The car headed for Suitland Parkway, which would have put us in the direction of GW, still a good fifteen-to-twenty-minute drive away, depending on the late-afternoon traffic. Spotting a firehouse, we both concluded I wasn't going to make it if we didn't stop there.

The car slammed into the drive on Irving Street. I recall my head being jerked backward. Mike threw the gearshift into park and leaped out in one sudden swoop. He raced toward the red brick building, leaving the driver's door open and the motor running.

"I need some help. I've got Bruce Johnson out there, and he's having a heart attack." I could hear him shouting at two people in blue uniforms who had probably already seen their share of life-or-death situations. Heart attacks probably run a distant third to assaults and killings in this part of town.

The fact is, few African-American men anywhere survive the ride to a hospital after having a heart attack. But then, a heart attack for a forty-two-year-old man of any color was still rare.

The paramedics seemed to be processing the information. They strolled out to the car with a stretcher, and once they looked inside and saw me, their demeanor changed. It was as if they thought, *Damn, it really is one of those TV guys.* They stepped it up after that. I should point out that had my attack come a few years later, I would have been out of luck because by then that firehouse was closed due to city budget cuts.

The paramedics didn't ask where I wanted to go, or if I had insurance. Most of the patients they transport are not covered. I wondered as I lay there if it really made a difference. With sirens wailing and lights flashing, they rushed me to—where else?—Greater Southeast Community Hospital, which was a couple of minutes away.

My pain subsided. Maybe the paramedic had given me nitroglycerin. I really can't remember. "Forty-two-year-old black male, probable heart attack," she reported over the radio.

The ambulance raced back in the direction Mike and I had already covered: Stanton Road, Alabama Avenue to Southern Avenue. . . . Mike was trailing us in the news car and somehow retained enough composure to do what he had been trained to do: report the story. Keeping his right arm on the steering wheel, he used his left hand to videotape the moving scenes with a 35-pound video camera. Later, he didn't remember doing it. News people—we really are peculiar.

*   *   *

I had arrived in Washington in 1976 as the youngest reporter ever hired by then-WTOP-TV, which today is WUSA-TV9, a CBS affiliate. I was twenty-five, with a wife and a toddler daughter. I had no health concerns, just a single job concern: to become the best broadcast journalist I could be.

My work was more than a career. It was a vocation, and it didn't scare me that I was arriving in the big city nearly broke, earning but $15,000 a year, slightly more than at my first job in Cincinnati at WCPO-TV. I would have come for less.

Getting to the nation's capital was the kind of opportunity my family members back home in Louisville, Kentucky, just didn't get that often.

In fact, I was the first, so my mom and seven siblings were both proud and afraid for me. D.C. was a long way from the Cotter Homes housing projects where we started.

In Cincinnati I had completed work on my undergraduate and graduate degrees. Those helped get me to D.C., but once I arrived, on-the-job training kept me there. A lot of smart people don't make it and get fired in this business because they're not quick studies, can't handle the competition or the stress of deadlines. I had to learn quickly, or I was going to be sent packing. By the time I arrived, WUSA was the No. 1 station in town; sometimes its newscast audiences were double those of the nearest competitor.

The station was headed by legendary news director Jim Snyder. He hired me based more on a hunch than on my videotape resume. I wasn't sure why they even needed me. The team already included established news anchors Max Robinson, Gordon Peterson, Maureen Bunyan, JC Hayward, and eventually sports anchor Glen Brenner.

Veteran WUSA reporters like Mike Buchanan, Pat Collins, Andrea Mitchell, Bob Strickland, Patrick McGrath, Susan King, and Henry Tennenbaum were already top-shelf broadcasters. My job would be to bring energy, enthusiasm, and some investigative skills to cover the city streets and D.C. government. I would have to get better quickly. I did.

My baptism in Washington television came within a few months of my start. An armed group of terrorists took over three downtown buildings. The gunmen turned out to be Hanafi Muslims, and they were making several outrageous demands. They wanted the government to hand over the men who had been convicted of killing seven relatives—mostly children—of Hanafi leader Hamaas Khaalis.

It was a religious feud. Three people were killed in the takeover. One of them was my friend and colleague Maurice Williams, a twenty-four-year-old reporter for Howard University's radio station, WHUR. One of the Hanafis shot him point blank as he stepped out of a fifth-floor elevator in the District Building (City Hall). The Hanafis then shot a D.C. government special police officer, Mack Cantrell, as he was responding to the earlier gunfire. Mack later died of a heart attack while recovering in the hospital. Marion Barry, then a city councilman and later mayor, was also shot and wounded. He managed to stumble into the council chambers, where other legislators and their staffs were beginning to bar the doors and flip over tables to use as cover from the armed terrorists.

For two and a half days, under nerve-wracking and dangerous conditions, I and other reporters worked round the clock covering the story. It was the first time I had ever done live shots, which meant standing in front of a camera—with hundreds of thousands of viewers at home—explaining, often with no script or notes, what was going on while the story changed by the minute. "Shots have been fired inside the building, but it's impossible to determine who was shooting and whether there have been casualties." We had to fill a lot of air time, which often meant recapping or repeating the same information again and again.

There was no time to be afraid or nervous. Hell, there was little time to eat. I recall telling viewers in one live report, just minutes after learning it from police sources, that "trapped city workers are now being escorted down fire department ladders that stretch to the fifth-floor windows in the back of the building."

Channel 9's ratings went through the roof. Max Robinson's anchor work for the story turned out to be an audition for the ABC network, which eventually hired him as an evening news anchor from Chicago. Max became the first African-American anchor on network TV.

By the time my heart attack hit me, I had become a veteran street reporter and weekend anchor with a boatload of Emmy Awards in my trophy case, and I was still fishing for more.

*   *   *

On the day of my heart attack, I was on what I thought to be a routine assignment in Southeast D.C. We were hoping to make a story out of Mayor Sharon Pratt's summer-jobs program for local youths.

"If we can just get these kids some kind of work," the program director said, she was sure they would stay away from drugs and the notoriously dangerous neighborhood streets. I agreed but didn't think a summer-jobs program was a big enough incentive. Back in Louisville, two of my brothers had sold drugs and eventually were arrested and sent to prison.

The location was East Capitol Dwellings, the city's largest public-housing project, so big that it expanded into both the Northeast and

Southeast quadrants of the District of Columbia. City officials would eventually give up on rehabilitating the place, instead tearing it down and replacing it with smaller and fewer detached, market-rate housing units.

My attention was drawn away from the long line of summer-job applicants at the community center to four young males watching, mockingly, from a distance.

In exchange for their interviews, I agreed not to reveal names and faces; then with camera rolling, they boasted that they already had gainful employment, albeit illegal. They were East Capitol Dwellings drug boys, fourteen, fifteen, and sixteen years old, who claimed to be earning hundreds of dollars a day selling reefer or crack.

I never believed the pay. They were exaggerating for the camera—and one another—but it was their story, not mine. What couldn't be hyped was the danger that surrounded their occupation. The drug boys proudly pulled up their shirts, eager to show off the long surgical marks from gunshot wounds to their abdomens. To them, these were battle scars, the cost of doing business on the streets. Those who survived multiple shootings earned immediate street credibility. Those who died got their sneakers tied together and tossed into the air until they draped over the telephone lines as lasting tribute to the fallen.

*   *   *

The doors swung open as I was rolled into the emergency room at Greater Southeast Community Hospital. Before, I had been here chasing ambulances with gunshot victims from the surrounding neighborhoods, maybe even one of those young men I had met minutes before on the street corner. What I now saw startled me. Doctors shouted orders, nurses scrambled to comply. Several sets of hands were all over me. Someone was cutting off my clothes. It was a good suit. *Why*, I wondered, *were they so sure I wouldn't need it again?* Someone put an IV needle in my arm, while someone else pasted leads on my chest that led to a telemetry machine monitoring my heart. I heard the blips the machine made and an occasional alarm when my heart skipped a beat.

An emergency room physician, Dr. Kenneth Larson, said when I spoke to him later, "You came in in severe pain. You were very, very upset that something awful was happening to you. You knew you were sick. I think you suspected that you were having a heart attack, but you didn't want to know it."

There seemed to be so many people milling around—a lot for the middle of the day in an ER. Was I the only sick patient here? I was given oxygen. My blood pressure and heart rhythm were taken. A second electrocardiogram seemed to confirm a big problem, although no one told me at the time. It didn't seem to be any of my business—saving my life! I was given a thrombolytic, or clot-busting, drug. I lost track of the pain and wasn't sure if that was because of the medication or a sense of dissociation. It was almost as if I had left the room. At some point Dr. Joseph Robinson appeared. He was whispering, checking the entire room, and I knew immediately that this was the guy in charge.

Dr. Robinson was the chief of cardiology at Greater Southeast. He's no longer there, and the hospital, after years of decline, was eventually bought by a private company that got millions of dollars from the D.C. government to close the deal. Without the cash infusion, Greater Southeast would have been taken off life support and eventually closed, leaving the entire area east of the Anacostia River without a hospital of any kind.

Dr. Robinson's day had been routine until I showed up. He remembers it this way:

I was in my office near the ER when I got the call from my ICU colleague that we had a VIP in the ER with an acute coronary event. Greater Southeast was not the kind of place that had many VIP's so I was curious. As always my mind was thinking through our protocol for heart attacks: diagnose, administer thrombolytic or clot-buster therapy, and stabilize. When I looked at the EKG strip the nurse gave me, I knew we had a serious problem. When she told me the patient was just forty-two years old, my concern grew. Bruce had the type of heart attack that has been called "the widow maker." Fifty percent of these patients die before ever getting to the hospital. Of the remaining fifty percent, another half doesn't make it no matter how well they are treated.

I didn't have to ask which bed Bruce was in; the noise behind the curtain was the giveaway. Didn't anybody tell them the last thing heart-attack patients need is excitement? I poked my head around the curtain and saw half of Channel 9 surrounding a man I recognized as the normally confident reporter I was used to welcoming into my home. But the man I saw was clearly as nervous as he could be. Bruce had the look associated with the word "doom."

I stood there with my arms folded and introduced myself. There was silence, and everyone simply evaporated. I remember Bruce's first words to me: "You must be important. Am I dying?"

"Sir," I said, "you've certainly had a massive heart attack, but I'm here now, and I've been doing this a long time, and my patients don't die." It was a white lie, of course but it was the right thing to say.

I'm not sure if I ever believed everything Dr. Robinson told me. I always had a healthy mistrust of anyone in authority, including doctors. But I knew my life had slipped out of my hands, and that I was going to get through this only if God wanted me to, so I surrendered then and there. I didn't want to die, but if it was going to happen, no one would say I went kicking and screaming.

I thought, *Would there be a life after death?* I grew up Catholic and believed so, most of the time. What a scoop to learn the answer to one of life's greatest mysteries. Maybe I would soon be seeing my younger brother David, my Great-Great-Grandma Millie, and even my natural father, who had all passed away. As I lay there I again became the child who needed to talk to God the Father whom I first met at Immaculate Heart of Mary grade school in Louisville.

A long, empty, silent corridor appeared before me. I strolled down it slowly, focused on the glowing light at its dead end. There was a door to the right. Should I turn right, or left, away from the door? I took my time making a decision. I chose not to enter the door and turned left. It was the right decision. I woke up, still in the ER. To this day I am not sure if it was a near-death experience or the drugs given me in the ER.

*   *   *

At the time of my heart attack, I was married to Madge, the mother of my two children, Kurshanna and Brandon. Madge had rushed to the hospital from Montgomery Blair High School in Silver Spring, Maryland, where she taught home economics. The only times either of us had been in a hospital were the births of our children. Madge recalls:

> *You were Superman, and nothing could harm you or stop you from doing whatever you wanted to do. I couldn't understand why this was happening. My heart was beating so fast. I just froze when I saw you in the hospital bed, helpless and fragile.*

If Madge ever thought I was going to die, she never said as much. Neither of us wanted to go there.

Dr. Robinson pulled her aside and tossed a barrage of questions her way. Did I have any medical conditions? Did I use drugs? What about cocaine?

"No, never," she said. I had smoked pot occasionally in college, and once dropped a half tab of LSD for the thrill. While still in college, I picked up a cigarette once in a while, and I became a full-time smoker while a reporter-in-training in Cincinnati. Back then nearly every veteran journalist had a cigarette in his mouth and, when possible, a stiff drink in his hand. I had dropped the Benson and Hedges pack-a-day habit a good year before my heart attack. A hypnotist helped me quit. My heavy drinking stopped two years before my heart attack, after I voluntarily entered an outpatient alcohol-rehabilitation program that Suburban Hospital ran in nearby Rockville, Maryland.

Only Madge knew that. I had kept my rehab secret from my TV bosses, friends, and family back home. I paid in cash for the six-week counseling sessions because I was afraid of having my health insurance company know. I never picked up another drink or cigarette after I quit.

Did I get clean too late? Part of me was thinking, *I have colleagues who smoke more and continue to abuse booze and drugs, but they aren't here on their backs.* Another part of me was thinking, *I brought this on myself with my reckless lifestyle up until a few years ago.* I was resenting my heart attack while at the same time feeling I had no one else to blame.

My closest friend at Channel 9, Gordon Peterson, arrived in the ER when he should have been back at the station preparing to anchor the six o'clock newscast. I told Gordon I was surprised to see him. "I didn't even think you knew how to get over to this poor side of town." We both laughed, a little.

Meanwhile, Mike Fox was huddled outside the ER punishing himself. He would later tell me, "I just ignored your symptoms. I figured if you were sick you would tell me." He eventually confessed that when he was eleven or twelve, he witnessed his father being carried out of their home suffering from a heart attack.

That night at the hospital, after everyone had left but my immediate nursing staff, the chest pain came back with a vengeance. By telephone, Dr. Robinson made the decision to have me transferred to the Washington Hospital Center. *U.S. News & World Report* says it's in the top twenty when it comes to heart centers in the country. The decision was OK by me. Two of my nurses brushed back tears. One of them grabbed my hand and practically apologized that Greater Southeast couldn't do more for me.

"We need to do a rescue angioplasty," Dr. Robinson told me, "and we'll need surgical backup in case we have to open you up." Then he added, "You'll be transported by helicopter."

"Will you be with me?" I asked.

"I don't do helicopters, they're too dangerous."

I don't remember much about the ride aboard the MedStar helicopter. My mind was in a fog. I do remember that there was a beautiful, clear night sky, and that the stars twinkled through the window of the chopper. Is that the Capitol dome down there below us, or am I just imagining it?

The Washington Hospital Center is on Irving Street in Northwest, just off North Capitol Street. That's a short distance from the Capitol to the south and the National Catholic Shrine a couple of blocks to the east. It's easily the area's premier heart-care center, with more than eight thousand catheterizations and one thousand five hundred open-heart surgeries performed there each year.

I recall Dr. Robinson was already in the cath lab and wearing blue scrubs when I was rolled in. Dr. Louis Kanda, a noted cardiac surgeon who bore an incredible resemblance to actor Sidney Poitier, was also there. Dr. Kanda has performed thousands of heart surgeries at the center and in faraway places like Africa and the Philippines. He would later say that as a generalization, he could tell if he was working on a black or a white man by the condition of the heart he held in his hand. Blacks always seemed to get to the emergency room with more heart damage. It was part economic, he said, but it also had to do with waiting too long to act, ignoring the symptoms of a heart attack when lives could be saved. Dr. Kanda was standing by in case multiple-bypass surgery was needed to try to save my life. Then there was Dr. Hector Collison, one of the busiest and most-sought-after cardiologists in the Washington area. He would eventually preside over a dozen separate practices in D.C., Maryland, and Virginia. On this early morning, he would preside over my emergency treatment.

I was placed on a table with an X-ray machine above me. There was another IV. I was hooked up to an electrocardiogram and other machines that kept track of my pulse, blood pressure, and other vital signs. A catheter, or thin plastic tube, was then inserted through an incision in my groin to a major artery. The catheter was threaded over a guide wire (which was removed once the plastic tube was in the artery), then into my coronary arteries and, finally, the heart chambers. A dye was injected to provide images for the X-ray machine.

The procedure, known as an angiogram, allowed Drs. Collison and Robinson to identify the blockages that were causing my pain and determine how much, if any, heart-muscle damage had occurred. I was awake the whole time and was actually encouraged to watch the incredible process through a monitor attached to a tiny camera that panned my sick arteries.

It didn't seem to take long before they thought they had detected my problem, my would-be killer: a soft clot blocking my left anterior descending coronary artery. The next step would be angioplasty. A wire with a tiny compressed balloon wrapped around its tip was threaded up to my heart from the same femoral artery in my groin. The wire broke though the soft plaque, and the balloon was decompressed. The wall of the artery was clear, and my blood vessel was wide open again. The balloon angioplasty was a success.

"If your pain was 10 when we started, what is it now?" Dr. Robinson asked.

"Zero," I said, but I wasn't sure of anything. This seemed like an out-of-body experience.

"That was the easy part," he said. "Now we have to find out why it happened in the first place, and how to prevent it from happening again."

Drs. Collison and Robinson chose not to insert a stent to help keep the artery open, a practice that would eventually become widespread, although not without its complications. They would monitor my damaged artery closely for restenosis, or reclosing, which happens to a number of patients' opened arteries, sometimes hours or days after angioplasty.

I wasn't out of the woods. There had been significant damage to my heart. A lower part of the muscle wasn't doing its job—helping pump blood. It would be weeks before I was out of acute danger, and it would take years before I was able to mend much of my broken heart and accept the events that transpired that day. I came to realize that admitting I had had a heart attack and accepting that I nearly died were two different things, the latter being more difficult.

I was in intensive care for several days, flat on my back because of the incision in my groin where Dr. Collison had threaded the wire through my femoral artery to my heart. There was good reason for the doctors to keep me still, with a weight putting pressure on the top of my leg, as any bleeding in this area could be fatal.

"You were the best patient," said Beverly Moncrief, my favorite nurse in recovery. I hit her with every question that came into my head. When would I know I had turned the corner? Is there something the doctors are not telling me? Every day was a press conference between us. Beverly would give me answers in her thick Jamaican accent, but never anything that should be coming from Dr. Robinson. She tried to keep me calm and confident, but she also wanted me to know that I was still very ill. When my despair crept into our talks, she would sometimes try to steer the conversation to another subject, spilling intimate details about her own close family. I felt at times that Beverly and the staff at Washington Hospital Center had become a part of my family.

I was always afraid of how this would affect my children. No father wants his kids to see him sick and laid up in a hospital suffering from a heart attack; that's what happens to old men, not me. They would need help getting through this as well.

Kurshanna was seventeen and a senior at Wilson Senior High School. Her mother broke the news to her as she returned home from a part-time job. Here's how Kurshanna recalled that day:

It was July 2, and I was returning home from my first "real" summer job, interning at the U.S. Senate Computer Center. As I was walking down the street, I could hear Dad's car driving up as it did every evening around 6:30 p.m., but this evening was different. Mom was getting out of the car instead of Dad. She always complained about Dad's car being too big for her to drive, so I found it strange that she had it and asked, "What did you do, kill Dad and throw him in the trunk. Why are you driving his car?" Boy, she looked at me funny but didn't say anything right away.

Personally, I thought my joke was funny until she mumbled the words, "Your dad has suffered a heart attack while out on a story. He is in the hospital right now." Immediately I lost all feeling in my legs and couldn't hear a sound. It was like the Earth stopped and I was the only one left to face reality. I finally managed to whisper, "What?" In my head I was screaming, kicking and crying, but nothing left my mouth. I simply could not move. It felt like I stood outside for eternity. To this day I still don't know how I walked into the house.

My 12-year-old son, Brandon, was finishing up a week at Art Monk's football camp in Western Maryland. It was his second year in the program run by the Redskins Hall of Fame player. I was going to miss the big intersquad game set for the final day, and I made sure no one put a scare into him or a damper on his camp experience with my bad news. I made the decision not to tell him until after camp had ended that day.

Kevin King, a cameraman and another good friend, picked my boy up from camp. Madge later brought Brandon and Kurshanna to the hospital. My son would later write:

> As I walked in the room cautiously I saw my dad, Superman, lying in the bed. Between the beeps of the monitors and the IV tubes, I really didn't have a reaction. The look on my face probably said it all. I remember him saying, "It's OK, you can cry," and I fell to pieces. . . . The rest of the visit is a blur for me.

When my children appeared in the doorway of my hospital room, it seemed like weeks since I had last seen and held them. "I'm OK," I said, knowing they needed to hear those words from me and not Madge or the doctor.

I took my first steps after about a week—or did it just seem that long? It was a Sunday, and I could hear a Sunday morning gospel program on another patient's radio. The host was Patrick Ellis, a fixture on WHUR-FM for years. "And this next song goes out to brother Bruce Johnson, who is recovering from an illness at the Washington Hospital Center. We wish you all the best, Bruce." I was surprised that anyone on radio would know about my predicament. I must admit I didn't like hearing my situation described as "an illness." I was too young to be ill. I almost wish I'd been shot, like those drug boys in Southeast. Old people get ill. Young people get shot. How sick is that?

Mayor Pratt called me. Assistant Police Chief Ike Fulwood stopped by. Former Redskins defensive back Brig Owens came to visit. Every member of the D.C. City Council checked in or sent cards and flowers. The city's delegate to Congress, Eleanor Holmes Norton, sent a personal message.

By the middle of the second week, at least half of the Channel 9 newsroom had shown up at my room. TV viewers filled my cardiac-unit suite and my home in Northwest D.C. with flowers and gifts. York Flowers on Wisconsin Avenue in Upper Northwest made a small fortune from my heart attack. Local bookstores also did well. Joan Gartlan, one of my reporter colleagues, brought me my first John Grisham book, *A Time to Kill*.

War, the singing group that recorded *All Day Music, The World Is a Ghetto, Cisco Kid,* and *Low Rider,* sent me a personal video. I had interviewed them at Washington's renowned Blue's Alley Jazz club.

All the while, doctors were coming by to examine my bed chart. "What do you think?" I recall asking one who seemed to ponder the information longer than the others. "Well, I've seen it go both ways," he said. "I've seen patients survive who took this kind of hit, and I've seen the others . . ." His voice trailed off.

I often felt both grateful and guilty: grateful for having been spared, but guilty knowing that other people had second heart attacks and died right there in the hospital. I wondered if I should bring in my attorney and draw up a better will.

My mom came. She flew in the day after my heart attack and wouldn't leave my bedside. She took my calls and screened my visitors and explained that she was so needed she wouldn't be returning to Louisville any time soon. For her own reasons, my mother was convinced that only she was capable of caring for me. We had already been through so much together, just the two of us, in the month before my heart attack.

* * *

Ma, that's what we called her. Mary Johnson Marbry was her name. Ma had been visiting us in June 1992, along with Madge's parents and her two sisters. Kurshanna was graduating from Wilson High, and Brandon was completing sixth grade at nearby Shepherd Elementary. Education was always celebrated in our families. I was the first to complete college; four of my seven siblings followed over the years, and my mother had earned her degree from the University of Louisville when she was fifty-two.

So for this double graduation weekend, not only was my mother visiting, but she brought my nephew Phillip along. Actually, Ma was peeved because she had wanted more of her family to be there, but Madge's people had reserved space first at the house. Kurshanna was the first grandchild and first niece in their family, and they had shown a special interest from the beginning.

How this weighed into my mother's decision to reveal her long-held secret I don't know, but I'm convinced it was a factor. I think she saw Madge's family filling a void in my life, the life she had created but, more importantly, had been unable to create: a two-parent household, as opposed to the stereotypical single black woman head of the house.

On June 19, after the graduations were over, I was sitting alone at the breakfast table reading a newspaper with my mandatory first cup of coffee. I grind the beans myself. This was before Starbucks was on every corner. I was the only one who could make the java strong enough but not too bitter.

Ma came around from where she had been tidying the kitchen counters and sat down across from me. She started mumbling in a soft voice, almost as if speaking to herself.

"Your father died two years ago."

"What?" I said, only half listening. My ritual of reading the paper before leaving for work isn't a luxury. It's my job; it helps me know what's going on in the city, and where I might find some leads to follow up. I hate it when my mother or anyone else interrupts my homework assignment.

"I said your father died, and I brought the obit with me from Louisville." I stopped and looked up because I sensed there was something very wrong in the works.

"What did you say? You mean Les? I thought he was dead already?" Les was my mother's first husband and the father of my brothers—Les, Michael, and David—and, I thought, me. Ma divorced Les and later married James Marbry. They had four children: Phillip, Ordette, Don, and Doug.

"Les was not your father. Your real father was Robert Richard Marshall."

She told me I was the result of an affair during a time when Les had abandoned her. So I have three sets of stepbrothers and sisters, including Robert Richard Marshall's children. It turns out Bruce Johnson is a bastard. On that day in June it was hello-goodbye to the father I never knew and would have no way of knowing. He had died, and my mother said he never even knew I existed.

I promised myself that if I survived the heart attack I was going to Louisville and learn all I could about Robert Richard Marshall. The results, I could never have imagined. Years later his children welcomed me, and even his widow insisted on meeting me. Surprisingly, I look more like our natural father than either of his other two sons. My stepsiblings were stunned by the resemblance. Ma couldn't have guessed that by revealing the secret she had kept to herself all those years we would become closer, but that's what happened after some tears and lots more questions and answers. I had become as interesting as some of the stories I covered as a reporter.

* * *

Now my immediate assignment was learning why I had had a heart attack and what I could do on my own to prevent another one. If I ever got out of this place, I didn't want to come back.

From literature within reach of my bed I read again, probably for the first time since grade school, that the four valves in my heart open and shut with precise timing like one-way doors to keep the blood flowing in the proper direction. The sound created by the closure of the valves is the heart beat, and each time my heart pumps or contracts, blood from the left ventricle moves out into my arteries. What I really wanted to know was who or what decides when the heart starts and stops?

Looking back, I had done my part to push my organ to the brink. A poor diet of red meats, starches, and fat helped propel my cholesterol into the stratosphere—nearly three hundred. That alone could help explain the clot that stopped my blood flow. I surmised that my heart had faltered like a bad piston under the car's hood and was no longer capable of supplying my brain and body with blood, oxygen, and nutrients. If I was going to get back out there on the road, I was either going to have to fully restore my heart functions, or at least rebuild and make the best use of this broken heart.

I needed some new tools. What had worked for me in the past would no longer do. On my own, I somehow rediscovered prayer and meditation while still in the hospital. This would help me cope with the stress. It had been years since I got down on my knees to pray; they just couldn't bend in that direction anymore. That also changed with practice.

Dr. Robinson convinced me that just as a brief rehab program had helped me stop drinking, a cardiac-rehab program could help me stop abusing my heart, while I also made some lifestyle changes.

At Greater Southeast, Dr. Robinson had developed a cardiac program that focused on prevention and rehabilitation. His innovations included hypertension clinics at barber shops and a walking program for men and women at nearby Iverson Mall before the stores opened.

The Washington Hospital Center had a very good rehab program. But I don't think I ever saw another patient my age. They were all much older, at least sixty-five. I wanted to appear encouraged and enthusiastic, if only because I had been "outed." They knew who I was—that I was on TV; but I was only forty-two and very embarrassed for having to be there. I thought perhaps I should blame Robert Richard Marshall, the father I never knew, for giving me his DNA. But Anne Ackerman, the rehab head nurse, helped me accept my predicament if only temporarily. Holding resentments or feeling sorry for myself wasn't going to help me get better. Anne told me: "The power is in the story of one patient to another. They carry a story that the staff doesn't carry. We know the kinds of things you need to do to be healthy, but often the role model for you is someone who is sicker than you that's already made changes."

A mere two weeks after my middle-of-the-night arrival by helicopter at the Washington Hospital Center, I was walking—albeit very slowly— on a treadmill, rowing a machine, and pedaling a bike. It wasn't the kind of training that would qualify me for a marathon—or even a brisk walk—but it was a start. All the while I was attached to a heart monitor with a panic button nearby in case the staff had to sound a code blue alarm for a cardiac arrest. A rehab nurse routinely checked my blood pressure, pulse, and weight. "You need to know your numbers yourself," she told me. "They're yours." She reviewed my medications and then confirmed that I knew how to take them.

Two weeks after my heart attack I was sent home, and I continued my supervised cardiac rehab as an outpatient for six weeks. When I wasn't at the hospital I was at a local fitness club, where I worked out on my own. I had been an avid racquetball player, but I knew I wasn't going back there. I no longer trusted the sudden starts and stops; the energy bursts that were required scared me. Basketball and touch football were also out for the same reasons. I needed an activity that gave me more control of how my heart sped up. I missed the burn from tense competitive sports, but I didn't want the risk of having to respond to a competitor's moves. My new beginning would need a new activity that I could become passionate about. Running seemed to be a safe, logical choice. My initial motivation was that when I returned to work, I wanted to return looking physically fit, rested, and certainly not like I had been through a near-death experience.

At the Tenley Sport and Health Club, I started with a routine that included workouts four or five times a week: three miles on the treadmill, fifteen minutes on the weight machines, no heavy barbells, no bench pressing or lifting above the head. No pressure on the chest. I listened to my body for any troubling signs, but I wasn't afraid to push myself, because I wore a heart monitor.

Eventually I was able to run three and a half or four miles, and my pace was improving: twelve-minute miles to start, then eleven, ten, nine, and eventually I was pushing eight-minute treadmill miles with a steady pace. If someone was on the treadmill beside me, young or old, I used it as a competition. The machines were working. The abs and shoulders were showing definition. I hadn't looked or felt this good in many years.

My diet had become one of low-fat foods, fruits and vegetables, broiled fish and chicken, skim milk, juices, and no soft drinks. My favorite snack was hot-air popcorn with Pam cooking spray, an artificial butter called Molly McButter, and light salt. I once complained about boredom with foods to my nutritionist after passing on a few spare ribs at a picnic. She explained that I should have sampled the ribs. "Moderation is the key, Bruce, not total denial," she said.

I moved my runs outside to Rock Creek Park, near my home. I could sense my heart getting stronger. Five workouts a week will do that.

I walked back into Channel 9 TV two months after suffering my heart attack on the job. My colleagues gave me a standing ovation. "Thank you. Thank you." The words came out effortlessly. I meant them. It was good to be back, to be part of the team, and to earn my keep. My first report after returning aired that very night. It was an exclusive story. The kid was back.

Dr. Robinson became as much a friend as he was a great doctor. We both had sons. We belonged to the same college fraternity, Kappa Alpha Psi. And we would eventually both get divorced. He insisted on performing every preventive or exploratory procedure available when it came to my heart. Over the next few years there would be echograms, treadmill stress tests, nuclear stress testing, and another catheterization, just to be safe and make sure the artery had not begun to close again.

I was brought back to the Washington Hospital Center, placed on another gurney, and had another slit made in my groin. I knew the drill. This time Dr. Robinson was presiding with a few nurses assisting. A wire with a tiny camera was again sent into the artery that had been closed by the clot. If the problem area had closed again, or any new closures were discovered, a tiny stent would be inserted to keep the artery open. It's done hundreds of times a month at WHC. It turned out that the artery that had betrayed me was still open. The patient was doing well. The doctor stapled my incision closed, and I was sent home after a couple of hours in recovery.

For months and eventually years, Dr. Robinson seemed almost stunned by my recovery. He called me a miracle, but I was never sure if he meant it or was setting me up for some bad news that might be lurking down the road. My ejection fraction was good. That's the measure of the percentage of blood that is being pumped out by both heart ventricles during the contraction, or pulsing, phase when both are at full capacity. If the EF is close to 55 or 60 percent, that's good. Mine was even better, and Dr. Robinson said all the credit was mine because of the great workout regime I had established. If my ejection fraction was well below 55, it would have been a sign that my damaged heart was not responding, and that eventual heart failure was possible.

"Continue what you've been doing would be my best advice," he said. He told me that a pacemaker might be advisable later. "It would be like a spare tire as you approach age 60. It's there if you ever need it, although you may never need it."

*   *   *

Someone once said, "If you want to just run, run a mile. If you want to experience another life, then run a marathon."

Under no circumstances would I have attempted to train to run long distances without my cardiologist's approval. No heart-attack survivor should attempt such strenuous exercises without his doctor's endorsement and the proper training under an experienced runner.

Running had become my passion, even more so than my TV work, and I decided I would run a marathon. Not because no other heart-attack survivor I knew had done so. I wanted to enter the Marine Corps

Marathon in Washington because few healthy people had ever run 26 miles, 385 yards. I needed to prove to myself that I was now healthy and whole. I had always been very competitive, and I still needed physical challenges.

I missed the online deadline for entering my first race in 1999, but I continued to train for another full year, entering small charity runs along the way to stay focused and tuned. I drove to the Marine base in Quantico, Virginia, the following year to register in person for the race in 2000. "It's certainly not something that I would do," Mike Fox said, while laughing through the telephone. "I guess you have to convince yourself that you are healthy again."

Dr. Robinson, in my last examination before the race, told me, "That heart can run in a marathon as long as you settle for just finishing and do not try and win the race." I would cling to his words. I should have put them on a T-shirt.

The vigorous training helped fill the void after Madge and I divorced following twenty years of marriage. Looking back, I realized I was often depressed after my heart attack, which I learned is common. It may have played a part in my decision to file for divorce, but it certainly wasn't the sole reason. Like all painful separations from someone you have been close to for a long time—in our case since college—it was like losing an arm and part of your heart. But my ex-wife and I agreed for our children's sake that we would always respect one another and our family after we went our separate ways. Madge and I remain friends today. I will always be grateful that she agreed to allow Brandon, who was entering ninth grade, to live with me. Kurshanna was a student at Howard University and living on campus at the time.

So the running came at a good time. It was my pause for reflection, meditation and prayer, my time to work on me. I ran the trails in the park. I ran in the streets. Beach Drive cuts through the center of Rock Creek Park from Rockville, Maryland, through Northwest D.C., where I live, all the way to downtown Washington alongside the Potomac River, past the Watergate Hotel and the Kennedy Center for the Performing Arts. I ran along the historic Chesapeake and Ohio canal to Georgetown.

My work schedule included anchoring the weekend newscasts, which helped me get long runs done on Thursdays and Fridays, my normal days off, and Saturday and Sunday mornings before I reported for work in the late afternoon.

I approached running like I approached my heart attack, first reading everything I could get my hands on, including *The Marathon: What it Takes to Go the Distance*, by Marc Bloom, *Making the Marathon Your Event*, by Richard Benyo, and *The Complete Runner*, by Bob Anderson. I worked my way up to a ten-miler, then a fifteen. The long-distance run was key, but I also added speed training, hills, and maintenance runs.

Famed marathoner Alberto Salazar once said "only dogs and wolves are as well-built for long distance running as humans." On my best days, I agreed with him. Interestingly, Salazar suffered his own heart attack well after his competitive racing career was over.

While I looked forward to most runs, there were times when I hurt and questioned whether my body—my heart—would fail me again. I sometimes stopped to check my pulse. I had become a master at picking up on anything out of the ordinary when it came to my body. Muscle pain was expected in the legs and arms after long runs. Cramps in the chest were reason to stop immediately and go through a checklist. I always carried identification that could easily be found and that made clear I had been a heart patient. I was always hydrated and seldom ran on an empty stomach, but never after a full meal. Once or twice there were long runs I could not finish and had to walk a remaining one or two miles home. And there were a few times when I questioned my sanity.

I used my Great-Grandma Millie, the daughter of slaves in Pembroke, Kentucky, as inspiration. I was running for Millie, who raised my mother and her younger brother in old wooden "shotgun houses" in Louisville's East End alleys. Ma told me during one of our long talks that they were evicted so often they sometimes didn't even bother to unpack when they first moved in. I was training and running for my six brothers and one sister back home in Louisville, and praying that they would always be safe from the drugs and violence.

I sometimes talked to my father, Robert Richard Marshall, even though I had never met him. "You would have been proud of me," I'd tell him. Never too old to play make-believe, I was running to be all that I could be, and when I wanted to quit I yelled out loud, sometimes cursing at myself, insisting that "quitting is not an option."

Runner Joe Henderson said, "Racing is a voluntary act of self-abuse. Before you decide to do it, you must be very sure this is what you want."

It's roughly nine miles from my front door to the other side of the Memorial Bridge that crosses the Potomac and takes you to Arlington National Cemetery. That's eighteen miles round-trip, the maximum run before I would compete in the Marine Corps Marathon. I made the big run twice before the October 22 event. My weekly total had surpassed seventy miles.

Other runners who knew my story were very encouraging.

"You walk through the water stations and run the rest of the way," advised Phil Fenty, the owner of Fleet Feet, a running store in the Adams Morgan neighborhood. Phil ran more than sixty marathons before retiring. Another marathon veteran, Mary Agnes Simons, a tough, rail-thin nurse, told me, "You won't even feel you are out there until about mile ten."

The morning of the race was cool. I boarded the subway, the Metro, with my girlfriend, Lori Smith, and we were met by scores of other runners who seemed to come from everywhere once we arrived at the parking lot of the Pentagon in Arlington, Virginia. We would board a shuttle that would take us to the Iwo Jima Memorial for the start of the race.

Lori had been a godsend in some of my toughest times. A single mother with a daughter, she stepped in to help with my son but never looked to replace his mom. She became a good friend to my daughter. She liked to run, so many days when I trained, Lori was there running alongside me, videotaping my form or waiting at the end of the road with encouragement. By October 2000, I was ready, twenty pounds lighter than when I'd had my heart attack.

My uniform consisted of black shorts, a blue sleeveless tank top with black trim, a white cap, black shades, and plenty of sunscreen. I had loaded up on carbohydrates the day before the marathon, tried to sleep that night, but couldn't. I hit the portable toilet like everyone else, and then waited confidently for the announcer to call my group out. My bib number was 3447—I'll keep it forever.

Lori and my kids would have to find me on their own after the race. I had no idea where I would end up.

Another well-known runner, John "The Penguin" Bingham, in *The Courage to Start*, wrote that "for all of us, the miracle isn't that we finish, the miracle is that we have the courage to start."

There were runners of all ages and sizes, and that was surprising. A few people were quite fat and appeared to be putting their hearts and joints at risk. About a quarter of the record crowd of twenty thousand appeared to be women. I was one of the few African-Americans.

The gun went off, and the race was under way. The real runners with Olympic speed were out front and engaged in their own competition. The rest of us laughed and yelled encouragement as we passed under the Marine Corps banner. I was determined to stick with a group that had vowed to run an average ten-and-a-half-minute mile. At the beginning we were one big mesh, moving at the speed of a camel . . . too many people.

We proceeded from the Iwo Jima Memorial through downtown Arlington, across the M Street Bridge, over the Potomac River, into the District of Columbia, through Georgetown, along Rock Creek Parkway on our way toward the Capitol. The TV station had assigned Mike Fox to videotape the race and me in particular. We ran past the Capitol, down the Mall to the Washington Monument, pointing toward Haines Point Park in Southwest. At mile ten, I was feeling a good burn in my legs. "Not so bad," I said out loud to no one in particular.

My original group had somehow disappeared. I fell in line behind other runners who were moving at a comfortable pace for me. I absorbed their energy, and they mine. As the race went on, the talk and happy chatter faded. Heavy breathing had taken hold of this crowd. Some of it was quiet and controlled; some of it loud and bothersome, unmasking the struggling runners who would eventually drop to the sidelines and quit.

By mile fifteen the race had become the grind everyone expected, and the cool morning temperatures were giving way to the noon heat. Earlier, when still fresh, I had passed my kids and friends, who waved signs and gave me high fives in the streets. Now I didn't want to see or hear them. *Just leave me alone to suffer and finish this*, I thought. I was hurting and couldn't fake another smile or fist pump if I wanted to.

At mile twenty, the water stations and tiny white cups that we had come to depend on had disappeared. I was dehydrated. My head and my hair hurt. The form was gone. My confident gallop had become a desperate stagger. I made it to the Fourteenth Street Bridge, where the toughest part of the marathon awaited me. It's called "The Wall," and it has nothing to do with the steep climb up the bridge. "The Wall" comes between miles eighteen and twenty, and it's when the body has used up all the carbs it could store, when much of the training and nutrition abruptly leave the body, and the runner is left to persevere through sheer will and mental toughness.

Everyone had warned me about "The Wall." I was now drained, exhausted, maybe even bordering delusional. A cramp suddenly struck a part of my leg and thigh where I had never experienced cramps before. I looked to my left and right. Other runners were also struggling. I lost track of the miles. The last few might as well have been another twenty. I knew it would eventually be over, but when? In minutes? Days? Amazingly, I never thought about my health, including my heart. I never thought I might have a second heart attack right there after crashing into "The Wall."

At the start of the race we had passed a runner who didn't survive. He was on his back, unconscious with an emergency medical technician standing between him and the rest of us so we couldn't surmise he had died. It had been his second marathon. News reports later said he was overweight and had barely trained for the marathon. I never worried. I had been at peace with my decision to do this. The rest was up to God.

Then, like someone stumbling in the desert and suddenly coming upon an oasis, I was almost there. The massive crowd at the finish line, maybe a half-mile off, was the giveaway. I slowed almost to a walk, but that hurt too much. I tried to pick up speed, but that hurt, too.

"Come on, Bruce, you can do it." Who was that? Out of nowhere I saw tiny Yvette Hess, a co-worker at Channel 9, who was watching the race from atop her bike. I continued up the hill back to the Iwo Jima Memorial.

I was done. I had finished. A young marine congratulated me while putting a medal around my neck and a silver wrap around my shoulders, designed to keep runners from going into shock. Mike Fox was at the finish line.

"How do you feel?" he asked.

"It's the hardest thing I have ever done," I told him.

This heart-attack survivor, now fifty years old, had completed the 25th Marine Corps Marathon. Wow! I felt great and awful at the same time. My time was four hours, thirty-six minutes, thirty-four seconds. I finished in the first half of all runners, and the first half of all runners in my age group. I was satisfied.

The marines helped me to the tent where my vital signs were checked. I overheard Mike tell them, "He had a heart attack a while back."

I was fine, but I could barely walk. My legs were saying, "We got you this far, the rest is up to your family and friends." Lori, Brandon, and Kurshanna helped me get to the shuttle bus and the subway. It was an awesome feeling. I never felt more alive than that day, never felt healthier. It's what a heart-attack survivor should feel every single day for the rest of their lives.

I continued my long-distance running five more years, until a bad hip pushed me to the sidelines. Then I bought a road bike. Today I continue to be physically active and still work as a reporter and anchor in Washington.

In December 2008, I underwent hip-replacement surgery, but I promised myself I would be back at work in roughly a month to cover Barack Obama's inauguration as the first African-American president of the United States in January 2009. I was out of the hospital in two days and back on the job in four weeks.

I helped cover the inauguration, working twelve- and thirteen-hour days at one stretch. I was on the air with good stories and memories to pass on to my children and grandchildren. I only wish Ma and Grandma Millie could have been there to see it. My mom had passed away two and a half years before from pancreatic cancer.

My heart continues to tick away years after my attack. I know that for some reason I was spared, and I continue to be grateful for this gift of life. My goal is to live each remaining day as though it's my last. Any day that I have been of service to someone else has been a good day for me.

Chapter 2:   Steve Sobelman

Dr. Steve Sobelman and his wife, Sloane Brown, sat relaxed in their fourth-floor apartment overlooking Baltimore's Inner Harbor.

Their place could be on the cover of *Living* or *Style* magazine. It's part of an old canning factory converted to condominiums. Olympic swimming super star Michael Phelps is one of their neighbors at the water's edge. Mystery writer Tom Clancy also lives nearby.

When you walk in, you're drawn through a narrow hall by natural light to the living room, which is surrounded by floor-to-ceiling windows looking south over the harbor toward historic Fort McHenry, where the British were stopped during the War of 1812 and Francis Scott Key wrote "The Star-Spangled Banner." The living room and kitchen are spotless, modern and bright. The den is dim and lined with photographs and hardcover books—the kind of den one would expect a noted college professor and an acclaimed newspaper reporter to have. A porch wraps around two sides of the living room and is overflowing with a jungle of well-kept plants. Though on the water, it's an urban place, and Sloane and Steve are urban people. Baltimore is where they work, play, and engage in a plethora of social and political activities.

Steve, a prominent psychologist in the Baltimore area, stands 6-foot-3 and has a cool, so-be-it attitude. Friends say he looks like movie mogul Steven Spielberg: he has the same salt-and-pepper back-combed hair, the same short-cropped beard, and the same rounded nose and bushy eyebrows.

Sloane is blond, elegant, and outspoken. She's the society and style reporter for the Baltimore Sun and writes columns on Sundays. What Sloane Brown writes, all of Baltimore's power players—the entrepreneurs, politicians, and civic leaders—are talking about

Between the two of them, Steve and Sloane seem to know everyone in town: politicians, ball players, political contributors. On the walls of their home are picture displays of them with prominent people who have passed through Baltimore. President Bill Clinton, Senator John Kerry—even Steven Spielberg. There's a picture of Steve and Sloane from the set of the 1988 film *Hairspray*. Neither is a trained actor; but they somehow managed to snag supporting roles in the movie, and they remain friends with its director, John Waters.

The couple is clearly living and thriving "in the moment."

"I'm a 'glass-is-half-full' kind of person," said Steve. "That's just who I am. It's never partly cloudy. It's always partly sunny."

Sloane is the same way. Worrying is a waste of energy, she said. Sloane lives by one of Steve's mantras: "As you think, so shall you be."

All that optimism was tested on a Sunday morning in summer 1992, when Steve suffered a heart attack, the kind that assaults the left side of the heart and often drops the victims where they stand, killing them in a matter of minutes. That was the kind that struck NBC-TV "Meet the Press" moderator Tim Russert in 2008 without warning while he recorded inserts for his popular Sunday talk show. And Army Command Sgt. Maj. Edward Barnett, killed by a coronary as he sat at his desk in Baghdad.

Steve first told me his story a year after his heart attack, not long after we had met and had both survived "the widow maker." The details were still fresh in his and Sloan's minds sixteen years later.

It started the night of June 5, at a baseball game at Camden Yards in downtown Baltimore. The Orioles were playing the Boston Red Sox, and Steve, Sloane, and a friend were watching from their seats on top of the third-base dugout. At one point, Steve got up to go for a beer. The short climb up the stairs to the concession stand left him gasping for air.

"God, I am so out of shape," he told his friend. "I am so out of breath."

Finally he was able to catch his breath. But that was strange, Steve thought. He wasn't *that* out of shape. After all, he exercised frequently and played organized sports. Maybe it was the humidity, he thought.

Steve went back to his seat and didn't give it another thought until they left the stadium after the game. That's when the shortness of breath hit him again like a punch right in the gut. Just walking to the train from the stadium had him gasping for air again.

"Steve was huffing and puffing as we were walking to the light rail," said Sloane, who found it curious but wasn't concerned. "I didn't think much of it," she said. "I was giving him shit about having to lose weight." At 240 pounds, Steve was overweight. In fact, he was the heaviest since Sloane had met him.

As they continued toward the train, Steve started to feel other strange sensations. He was now sweating, and pain that had started in his left shoulder was radiating down his left arm. "It was a numb pain, not shooting, but an internal numb pain," he explained.

This psychologist knew more than a few things about medicine. He was the chief of behavioral health at The Children's Hospital in Baltimore. He also knew more than the average Joe about heart disease: just a few years earlier he had helped set up the cardiac-rehab program at Children's Hospital.

The pain in his left arm was no longer a nuisance or mystery. Steve knew what it could mean. "Oh, shit," he thought. "This isn't good."

But in just a few seconds, the pain was gone. Heart attacks can come disguised at times. Even some of the smartest among us would rather rationalize a decision not to act rather than move quickly to seek emergency care or assurances that the pain is not being caused by a heart attack. Steve was no different. Although still concerned, he told himself he'd go to the hospital if the pain returned.

But while he procrastinated, the arteries supplying blood to the left side of his heart were being obstructed by plaque. Blood was coming through, but just a trickle. His heart was being deprived of oxygen-laden blood and was working furiously. He had no more pain that night. "When we got on the train, I was OK," he said. "And when we got home, I was basically OK. So I thought I was all right."

The next morning, a Sunday, Sloane left the house early to go shopping with her stepbrother. At the time, she and Steve lived in Lutherville, a suburb ten miles north of Baltimore. At about 11 a.m., Steve was helping his daughter's boyfriend on the computer. Suddenly the pain in his arm returned. He rushed into the bedroom, closed the door behind him, and sat on the edge of the bed. For no apparent reason he was sweating, just like the night before. He became nauseated.

But the worst part was the pain in his arm. It was worse than the previous night. It was terrible. "The pain in my left arm felt as though there was a vise on it, or a blood pressure cuff that someone just pumped up and never released," he said. "I felt nauseated, and I started sweating profusely."

There was no denying it now; Steve knew what all this meant. "Shit, I am having a heart attack," he thought.

For some god-awful reason, he still couldn't bring himself to reach for the phone to call 911 or yell out for help. "Sloane will be home soon," he thought. "Then we can go to the hospital."

Just then the phone rang.

"Hello."

It was his mother.

"How are you doing, Steve?" How do mothers always seem to know when something is wrong?

Steve didn't want to talk, and he certainly didn't want to alarm his mother. "I'm not feeling well. It's a little bug that's going around. I'll call you later."

Steve hung up the phone and fell back on the bed.

The pain continued, and Steve was scared. He took deep, steady breaths to control his breathing and calm himself. Then he focused on a leaf outside the window. He stared at it, not letting his mind wander back to the pain or the fear. This was self-hypnosis, a relaxation technique Steve used with some of his patients.

"I knew what was going on," he said.

In about twenty minutes, Sloane and Steve's daughter returned home.

"I really don't feel well," Steve told Sloane.

Sloane thought it was odd to see Steve in bed in the middle of the afternoon, but she wasn't convinced Steve was really sick. "I thought he was doing the typical guy thing when they don't feel well, which is, revert to infant status. I still thought he wanted attention."

"I think we should go to the hospital," Steve said.

"What's the matter?" Sloane asked.

"Little chest pains," Steve replied. He didn't have chest pains, but he knew this was a heart attack, and he wanted to get Sloane's attention. "Why don't we go to the hospital," he said again. "Why don't you drive?"

"OK," Sloane replied. "If you are really sick, we'll go."

Greater Baltimore Medical Center was the closest hospital, only a few miles away. The whole trip Steve was correcting Sloane's driving. "Turning left here?" he'd ask. "Make a right there!"

"Oh, yeah," Sloane thought. "You're having a heart attack, and you can still be a backseat driver."

At the emergency room lobby, Steve didn't waste any time. He went right to the triage desk. "I am having chest pains," he told them, using the same urgency he used on Sloane. "I think I am having a heart attack."

That was all the nurses needed to hear. They rushed Steve through the double doors into the bowels of the emergency room, where several teams were at work on several patients behind closed curtains.

Nurses hooked him up to an electrocardiogram to monitor his heart's electrical activity. He was feeling better again, and his heart wasn't showing any irregularity.

"Everything seemed to be fine," Steve said.

After a few minutes, the hospital staff brought Sloane back to see Steve. Suddenly, there was a shrieking noise: BEEEEEEEEEEEEP. It was the EKG machine, and it was going haywire. Sloane and Steve were both startled. What the heck did that mean? It sounded like an important alarm, but no one was rushing to Steve's aid.

"Finally," Sloane said, "a nurse ambled over and wiggled one of the leads, and the alarms stopped." It was nothing; Steve has a hairy chest, and one of the EKG leads had peeled free.

In a few minutes the doctor arrived, and he seemed unconcerned. "We might want to keep you overnight," he told Steve and Sloane. That was it. It didn't seem serious. Steve and Sloane chatted for the next few minutes, when all at once Steve felt sick again.

"I don't feel very good," he told her. "I feel sick to my stomach."

This time, Sloane didn't doubt it. She was standing over Steve, and he didn't look good. "You know," she told him, "you are looking a little gray."

Then things started moving fast. Suddenly, the EGK machine came alive again: BEEEEEEEEEEEEP. The noise must have been different this time, because doctors and nurses came running.

"There were a million people around me," said Steve, "and I am being wheeled down the hall."

"This time all these people descend on Steve," said Sloane, "and I was ushered out of the room. I knew now it was serious. They didn't want me there. All they said was, 'We need you to leave.'"

Sloane was pushed back to the waiting room. Meanwhile, Steve was writhing in pain as the staff rushed him to the operating room. "Crushing pain in the arm," Steve said later. "My arm was killing me."

"Can anybody do something to reduce the pain in my arm?" he screamed.

A moment later, Steve began to feel light-headed. "I think I am going to pass out," he told the staff. Doctors and nurse hovered over him. He could barely stay awake. "Steve, stay with us," the hospital staff kept screaming at him. "Stay with us! Just stay with us!"

* * *

Steve Sobelman had always been at high risk for cardiovascular disease and a heart attack. It was in his genes, and he knew it.

Born in the 1950s to first-generation Russian-American parents, Steve was raised in Morris Plains, New Jersey, twenty-two miles west of New York City.

"I grew up in a typical first-generation household," Steve said of his upbringing. "We ate heart-attack food: liver, bacon, meat, potatoes."

They also ate schmaltz, a Jewish spread made of rendered animal fat, made by Steve's grandmother who lived in a Russian immigrant neighborhood across the river in New York.

"She saved chicken fat and bacon fat and put it in a jar," Steve explained. "My grandmother would make great bread, and we'd slather that fat on the bread, and it always tasted good." Schmaltz is anything but health food. "Everything always tasted great, but it was never good for you," Steve said. "I'm surprised we didn't have heart attacks when we were eight years old." In those days, however, there wasn't the same concern about heart disease. "We never put that together," Steve said.

After high school, Steve entered Norwich University, a private military college in Vermont, where he studied English. One day during his senior year, Steve's mother called.

"Your father's fine," were her first words. Steve's mother was the dramatic type. She always had a handkerchief stuffed up her sleeve and would put it to her forehead in dramatic fashion.

"What do you mean?" Steve asked.

The day before, his father, a researcher for the Department of Defense, had given an address at Duke University. As he stepped off the stage, he complained that he didn't feel well, then collapsed. He was rushed across the street to Duke University Medical Center, where doctors discovered he'd had a heart attack. That was in 1967.

Steve was a bit shocked, because his father was physically active; he swam, golfed, and played tennis. "He was a pretty healthy guy," Steve said. "At least appearance-wise."

Steve caught the next plane for North Carolina to be with his parents. When he got to the hospital, there was Dad, pounding his chest defiantly. "Strong as a bull," he told Steve. "I don't know what happened. Just a little glitch. I'll be fine."

It was more than a little glitch. The attack severely damaged his heart, leaving only 25 percent of it working. He did, however, recover and live another thiry-plus years before dying of a stroke at eighty-three.

Steve was a young man when his father got sick, and therefore wasn't concerned about his own heart-health. "I thought, 'I'm pretty healthy, I'm an athlete, and I'm in pretty good shape.'" Steve said. "I didn't think anything could be wrong with me."

*　　*　　*

At Greater Baltimore Medical Center, the doctors saw that Steve was fading. He was losing consciousness and could hardly keep his eyes open. The clot in his coronary artery was starving his heart of the fuel it needed to work, and it was about to fail.

"Steve, stay with us! Just stay with us," the doctors screamed.

Steve could barely hear them. "OK, I'm trying."

Someone put an oxygen mask on his face. Then he heard the doctors talking about paddles. Oh, no, Steve thought, not the paddles.

Paddles are the nickname for the sandwich-size electrodes through which defibrillator machines deliver an electric jolt. The machines are used when the heart is in fibrillation, a state of irregular, rapid, or unsynchronized contraction. The shocks stop the heart momentarily, allowing it to restart itself with a normal rhythm. It's like rebooting a computer. Steve had seen doctors using defibrillators on television, and it didn't look comfortable for the patient. He also knew they were usually used in dire circumstances.

"That's odd," he thought to himself as they prepared the defibrillator. "Don't you have to be dead when they use the paddles?"

Before he was shocked, however, the doctors injected Steve with a strong dose of tissue plasminogen activator, or TPA, a clot-busting drug that, if given shortly after a heart attack, can dissolve the problem clots. Though effective, clot busters are powerful and potentially dangerous drugs. They can cause bleeding, and dosage errors can be deadly. That's why they are usually only administered in a hospital.

"It's working! It's working!" someone shouted. "And look! His vitals are coming up." They didn't need the paddles.

"It's like a Roto-Rooter," Steve said of the clot-busting drug. "And it goes right through your system, and all of a sudden the pain went away, and I felt better." But the drugs had thinned his blood so much that Steve's mouth was bloody. "Apparently I have weak little veins in my mouth." That was OK, though. "I was relieved because nobody was hitting me with paddles," he said.

It all happened so fast that Steve still didn't really know what was wrong to begin with.

"What's going on?" he asked the doctors.

"You were having a heart attack," they told him.

"Really?" he asked. "My arm was killing me."

*   *   *

Steve Sobelman got to Baltimore by way of American University in Washington, D.C., where he earned a Ph.D. in psychology. He took a job as a psychology professor at Loyola College, a Jesuit and liberal arts school in Baltimore, and eventually became director of graduate programs there. While also chief of behavioral health at The Children's Hospital, he started his own private psychology practice.

Steve has been married twice. He had two children, David and Stacey, with his first wife, whom he divorced in the early 1980s. In the early 1990s, he met Sloane in the newsroom at Channel 2 in Baltimore, where she was an anchor. Steve was there to be interviewed for a piece the station was doing on mental health. They were both single, and a cameraman set them up on a date.

Steve had always taken his health for granted, never really had to work at it. It was just part of his lifestyle. "I was very much into awareness . . . healthy body, healthy mind." And he was always searching for new health trends. He got into vitamins and started a daily regimen. He became a vegetarian a few times over the years, not because he didn't want to hurt animals but because it was a healthier lifestyle.

"But I was a novice with all [that] stuff," Steve said. "I sort of went with the fad as opposed to doing a lot of research."

And Steve had always been physically active. He could jog five miles, and he played basketball and fast-pitch softball. Lately, however, he hadn't been doing much cardiovascular exercise. "I exercised, but not the right way," he said. "I was lifting weights. I started to look portly."

"You were the heaviest you had ever been right before the heart attack," Sloane said. "Look at those pictures. He was really, really puffy. And I'm sure that had something to do with it."

"I never really thought there was anything wrong with me physically," he said.

*   *   *

Sloane doesn't remember how long she was in the waiting room after they took Steve away in a flurry of activity. All she knew was that he was in dire straits. She realized she was still holding Steve's glasses. "Oh, my God," she thought. "Is this the last thing I have of him?"

Finally, a nurse appeared. "Your husband is having a heart attack, and we are stabilizing him. He is going to be OK."

After that—it could have been many minutes or more—a group of nurses wheeled Steve past Sloane. He was on a gurney on his way to the cardiac intensive care unit, or ICU.

"I'm not feeling very well," he told her again.

Sloane tried to follow, but nurses stopped her and gave her directions to the ICU waiting room. Too much was happening too fast, however, and she couldn't concentrate. "The nurse ushered me to an elevator, and I stepped in and the door closed, and I turned to the people around me and said, 'I don't remember where I am going.'"

Sloane finally found the waiting room, and then the chief of cardiology appeared.

"I was flipping out, and he wanted to give me Cardiology 101 . . . explaining about the left side of the heart and blah, blah, blah."

Sloane was scared. "I wasn't interested in the intricacy of the heart. I just want to know how my husband is."

Then she got some information that she could process. Steve had had a heart attack, the cardiologist told her, and now they were stabilizing him and preparing for an angioplasty.

She wanted another opinion. Her reporter instincts said always get two sources when possible. She called a friend, Dr. Jeffrey Quartner, chief of cardiology at Sinai Hospital in Baltimore. Steve had worked with him at Children's Hospital.

Sloane found Dr. Quartner's number in a phone book and immediately went to a booth and called him at home. "I'll be right there," he told her.

When he arrived, he went right to Steve's bed. "Ah, this is just great. What you are doing here?" he joked. The doctor knew, however, that this was no joke. "We need to look at you," he said.

Steve was wheeled to the catheterization lab, where Dr. Quartner did an angiogram.

Steve was awake for the procedure and watched it on a video screen. "I found it interesting because I was watching what he was doing," Steve said. "He looked at the different arteries, checking for occlusion or blockage."

Sloane was watching, too. Her father was a doctor, and she had always been fascinated with medical procedures. "I saw all of Steve's blood vessels, and his heart pumping," she said. "It was really cool. It was neat." Both of them were clearly more relieved with someone they knew and trusted presiding over the procedure.

An hour after the angiogram, Dr. Quartner came to see Steve again. "You dodged a bullet," he told his old friend. "Your left anterior descending artery has no blood flow; only little drips are going through. It's 99 percent occluded."

In order to perform its job of pumping blood, the heart needs blood of its own, which it gets from the coronary arteries. Right coronary arteries supply blood to the right side of the heart, which receives deoxygenated blood from the body and pumps it to the lungs. The left coronary arteries, one of which is the left anterior descending artery, or LAD, supply blood to the left side of the heart, which receives oxygenated blood from the lungs and pumps it throughout the body. Because it pumps blood to the whole body, not just the lungs, the left side of the heart does most of the hard work.

Heart attacks occur when blood flow through a coronary artery is restricted or blocked, usually the result of a rupture of cholesterol and other substances called plaque. When blood flow is restricted, the part of the heart affected can be damaged or killed.

Left-side heart attacks like Steve's are the most dangerous type because that's the side of the muscle that fuels the whole body with blood. When one of the left coronary arteries is restricted, the left side isn't as efficient at pumping blood, resulting in symptoms like shortness of breath, sweating, weakness, and nausea. If the blockage is severe and not treated, blood stops flowing altogether. Loss of consciousness and death follow.

Dr. Quartner reminded Steve that this type of blockage is called "the widow maker."

"Healthy people can be walking down the street, and the next thing they know they just fall over dead," the doctor said. "If you had your heart attack any place else other than here, you would be dead. We wouldn't be talking."

When Sloane learned about the widow maker she realized how close she had come to losing her husband.

"If he had it at home, an ambulance could not have gotten to him in time," she said. "We were so lucky that he recognized the signs."

Because Steve's heart attack happened in the hospital, doctors were able to clear the clot almost immediately with the clot busters, so his heart wasn't without blood for long.

"I had no heart damage," Steve said. "We caught everything quickly. There was good karma going around."

Now that the problem was identified, they needed a permanent solution. Dr. Quartner told Steve there were three options: they could scrape his arteries clean, open them with angioplasty, or route his blood around the clogged artery with bypass surgery.

The doctor said bypass surgery would be the most effective. Steve trusted him and gave the go-ahead. He was taken by ambulance from Greater Baltimore Medical Center to Sinai Hospital, which had an advanced heart center, where he was scheduled for surgery the next morning.

Steve doesn't remember feeling scared before surgery. "I felt pretty confident that we were going to take care of whatever was wrong," he said. "I wasn't scared. I was a little numb to it. It all happened so fast. I am not aware that I was scared at all."

Dr. Quartner, however, saw the look on Steve's face. "You had that look that I see in a lot of patients," he told Steve later. "That wide-eyed, vacant look."

Sloane saw it, too. "You had a wide-eyed, scared look," she said.

"I never felt it," he said.

Sloane had held up well, but the night before surgery was particularly emotional. She was with Stacey, Steve's daughter, who had come to the hospital. "She came home with me, and I remember breaking down and really crying," Sloane said. "That night I absolutely was worried that I would lose my husband.... At times it was a huge emotional thing." That night, Sloane found comfort by sleeping in one of Steve's shirts.

The bypass surgery was performed in 1992. Dr. Quartner had brought in another skilled surgeon, Doctor Neal Salomon who would become the new director of The Heart Center at Sinai Hospital. Steve's body was cooled, which slows down the heart. Then doctors administered a solution called cardioplegia to stop his heart altogether so they could operate. A heart-and-lung machine took over the pumping and oxygenating of his blood. When the surgery was complete, Steve's heart was restarted in a procedure called reperfusion.

Later, the doctor told Steve, "I literally had your heart in my hands."

Steve awoke from the anesthesia to good news. "I was told that everything was successful," he said. And considering what he had been through, Steve felt pretty good. "After the operation, I felt fine," he said. "I was numbed up . . . [but] I felt good."

Sloane wanted to see Steve immediately, but the doctor warned that the sight of him could be overwhelming. "A lot of people get really freaked out because you're going to see all these tubes and wires going in and out of him," he told Sloane.

She wanted to see him anyway. He was semicomatose and on a ventilator. "I go in and, sure enough, there are wires and tubes going through his arms," Sloane said. She was fascinated by all the devices and high-tech equipment. "This is so cool," she said.

Then she started asking questions. "What's that for?" she wanted to know, excitedly pointing to a tube. That's cleaning his blood, the doctor explained.

"And what's that?" It was a Mylar blanket, the doctor told her. They had cooled Steve for the surgery and were now warming him back up.

"So it's like you are defrosting him."

"I don't think I've ever seen anyone react the way you reacted," the doctor told her.

Sloane explained. "I know that every single one of those things going in and out of my husband is for his good. I know that all of this is only to make things better for him, and I totally trust what you guys did. The more stuff there is like that, the better off he's going to be."

Sloane also wanted to know as much as she could about what was going on. "Knowledge is power," she said later. "The more I learned about what was going on, the more comfortable I got and the less scared I was. When they told me that the worst was over and they had him stabilized and this was routine, then I was able to calm down."

She also was able to put her trust in the doctors. "I forcefully believed in what the doctors were doing," she said. "I wasn't going to question it, and as a result I didn't go through all that catastrophising."

"He was going to be OK," she told herself.

The doctors were aggressive with Steve's recovery and encouraged him to get back on his feet as quickly as he could, even while he was still in the hospital. Steve took their advice, slowly walking the halls around his hospital room. As he passed other rooms, he'd glance inside at the other cardiac patients. "It seemed like I was the youngest one there," he said later.

Doing his rounds, Steve found himself transforming into doctor mode.

"How you doing?" he asked an older fellow.

"Oh, I had open-heart," the man responded.

"Me too. Come walk with me." Steve suggested.

The man didn't feel up to it. "I can't," he said.

But Steve didn't give up easily. "You've got to get up and running," he said. "Walking and moving. You just can't lie here, because you've got to be a good patient!"

Steve then told the man about the cardiac-rehab program he helped start at Children's Hospital. "I told him I wanted to get him in our program.... That's what we did; we got people after they had heart attacks or surgery. We'd get them in exercise programs, nutrition programs."

It wasn't all pain-free during those first few days, however. The worst part for Steve was something he never imagined: sneezing. "If you sneeze after you've had open-heart surgery, the pain just rattles through your body.... You think you are going to break apart. It wracks your whole body." Steve doesn't remember ever sneezing as much as he did after surgery. "All of a sudden, I was a sneezing fool," he said. "I'd feel a sneeze coming on and try anything not to sneeze."

All the staff could do for the sneezing pain was give Steve a heart-shaped pillow to hold against his chest to absorb some of his body's vibration. "I still have it," he said.

After two or three days, Steve was sent home with instructions to keep moving, to walk as much as he could. Within a week he was walking up to a mile around his neighborhood. He was feeling good, and his recovery was going as well.

"Guys like you make guys like me look great," Dr. Salomon told him.

But all that walking began to get tedious. And it was summer in Baltimore—so hot that even if you were in good health, you'd never want to go for a long walk outside. Steve started trying to skip his daily walks, but Sloane wouldn't allow it. If it's too hot to walk outside, she told him, they'll go to the mall and walk.

"I don't want to do that!" Steve shot back. Heat or no heat, walking outside was better than the mall.

"He could get a little cranky," Sloane said later.

Soon Steve started cardiac rehab—the same kind of program he helped start at Children's Hospital. He went three or four times a week, mostly riding the bikes and lifting light weights. He was feeling good, both physically and psychologically. Still, Dr. Solomon warned him that many patients experience post-heart attack depression.

"You don't know me," Steve told him. "I don't get depressed. That's just not who I am. I get tired, and down at times. Or just pissed off. But I see patients who are depressed, and I don't share any of what they bring to my office as part of what my life is about."

The doctors also wanted to give Steve drugs that would help his heart work with less effort and lower his cholesterol. But Steve didn't listen to them and didn't take the medication. "I wanted to do it naturally," he said of his recovery. "I wasn't taking any cholesterol-lowering drugs. I wasn't even taking an aspirin."

"Steve didn't go on any medication," Sloane said. "We were going to do it with diet, because he heard that things like Lipitor made you so tired."

The one piece of doctor's advice that Steve did follow had to do with exercise. "I went to the gym religiously," he said. "I was running, [doing] cardiac, getting the heart rate up and lifting weights."

And though his diet was never horrible, Steve started eating better food. It didn't take long before he had shed twenty-five pounds. He was now about 215. He also started taking lots of vitamins.

Between the bypass surgery and all that exercise, Steve was sure all his heart problems were in his past. "In my mind, I was totally clean," he said. I was like a newborn baby. I was feeling fine. I didn't feel any negative stuff anywhere."

But Steve was kidding himself. Yes, his diet and exercise had lowered his cholesterol, but it was still too high. And he still had heart disease—it was embedded in his genes.

And four years later, in 1996, it happened again.

Steve was in Florida for a few days visiting his parents. He was crawling around in their attic helping them wire the house for the Internet when he felt that familiar numbness in his arm.

"'Holy shit,' I thought to myself."

But again, like the last time, the pain went away as quickly as it had come.

"It was very hot [in the attic], and I attributed it to the heat," Steve said. "I didn't say anything."

Despite having such a close call four years earlier, Steve didn't rush to the hospital. The symptoms subsided, and he flew home to Baltimore the next day as scheduled. The next night, however, there it was again—that old familiar pain in his arm.

"You know what," he told Sloane, "I am starting to have these symptoms again."

At the time, Sloane was the entertainment reporter for Channel 7 in Washington, and the next morning, a Monday, she was due in New York for an interview. Steve planned to go along. Now, on Sunday night, he was feeling sick. But they weren't going to wait again. Sloane took him to the hospital. And when he got there, he went into cardiac arrest, just like the last time.

"I had another heart attack," Steve said. "It was on the right side. This time it was the right coronary artery."

Steve was shocked. For four years he had felt fine. He thought he was clean, clear, and healed. "Then, I'm back in the hospital." There was resentment, if not the outright anger most repeaters feel the second time.

This time doctors were able to clear Steve's blockage with a stent, but they told him he could have avoided the attack if he'd followed their advice and taken the medication. "You brought this on yourself. The exercise is great, but Steve, you have bad genes. This is all genetic. You may think you are Superman, but you are not."

"I got a big lecture from my doctor," Steve said.

Sloane and Stacey were at the hospital. They looked down at Steve in the bed, just where he had been four years earlier. The no-drug approach had failed. Not even exercise and a good diet had kept Steve's arteries clear. Sloane and Stacey decided that from then on, Steve would follow *all* the doctor's orders.

"You will now be taking any medications that Jeff says you should be on," Sloane told him.

Steve was released from the hospital the next day. And since then, he has taken all the medication the doctors have recommended.

"I take my Lipitor like everybody else," he said. "I take Zetia, Toprol, and I take Lotrel. And I take a baby aspirin. And then I take a bunch of vitamins." Steve also takes prescription niacin, a form of vitamin B, which increases the amount of good cholesterol, also called high-density lipoprotein, or HDL.

At first, the niacin made Steve sweaty and itchy, and he had hot flashes. It also turned his skin a reddish, flushed color. Then he switched to an over-the-counter form of the vitamin called no-flush niacin, which is less likely to cause side effects. The hot flashes ended, but Steve's skin still has a reddish hue.

"He tends to be very red," Sloane said. "Some people say, 'Wow, you've got a tan.' But no, he's just flushed. That's the niacin."

"I never used to blush," Steve said. "Now I blush at the drop of a hat."

The other medications have done their job. "My total cholesterol is 119. . . . My blood lipids are really good. . . . My glucose and triglycerides are good, too," Steve said. "That doesn't mean that I couldn't have a heart attack tomorrow, but . . . all my risk factors are low."

Steve used to feel a little embarrassed about having suffered a heart attack, as if it were some kind of weakness. Those feelings are gone now.

"I think it's kind of a badge of courage," he said. "And it's interesting. People want to know what it's like to go through that."

Steve also used to hate it when people saw the zipperlike scar over his chest from the open-heart surgery. Now he's more comfortable and says he sees himself as part of a club—"the Zipper Club."

One curious thing about Steve's heart attack, they both said, was the reaction of friends.

"They see themselves lying there," Sloane said of friends who visited Steve at the hospital. "That's what's really interesting. . . . It gives you a really interesting insight into your friends."

For some, it was emotionally jarring. "All of a sudden it made them very vulnerable and fearful," Sloane said. "A lot of them felt that this wasn't something they'd have to deal with for fifteen years or so."

One friend was particularly affected by seeing Steve. "You could tell he [wondered], *Could this happen to me?* [He wanted to know] how he could prevent it."

Another friend was too anxious to visit Steve in the hospital. Finally, Steve got him on the phone. "This isn't about you. It's about me," Steve told him.

Seeing his father so sick scared David, too. "I think it was probably more anxiety than anything else," Steve said. "He lost weight. . . . He was getting up to 250 or 260, and now he is down to 210, almost too thin."

Sloane and Steve handled Steve's heart disease with pragmatism and cool-headedness. Sometimes friends would ask Sloane, "Have you thought about what it would be like if he had died?"

"No," she'd reply, "because he didn't."

Steve heard the same kind of questions. "A lot of people ask, 'Was it life-changing?'" Steve said. "And it wasn't. We didn't go through the major emotional stuff that a lot of people do. I never said, 'Wow, I dodged a bullet and therefore I'm going to go to church every Sunday and thank God I am OK.'"

Others wanted to know if Steve's life flashed before his eyes. "It just didn't happen that way," he said.

Sloane thinks their strength has a lot to do with Steve's profession. "He is a really, really good shrink," she said. "And he taught me one of his mantras: As you think, so shall you be."

To Sloane, that means never letting her worrying get out of control and not catastrophising about what *could* happen. "It's a real waste of energy," she said. "You don't sit there and wonder about, *What if?* I didn't. Why put yourself through all that emotional baloney? Deal with what *is*."

Sloane uses the analogy of being stuck in a traffic jam—the same one Steve uses in his stress-management seminars. "If, when you are stuck in a traffic jam, you tell yourself, 'Now my day is going to be horrible, and my life is for shit because I am late,' then emotionally you find yourself getting really upset," Sloane explained. "You have an emotional reaction to how the situation is filtered through your own beliefs."

The key, she said, is beliefs. "If your own beliefs are, 'There is nothing I can do about this, and I will get to work when I get to work,' then you won't get so angry."

It's a technique that helped Sloane and Steve deal with heart disease. "We weren't going to sit there and start going off onto all these fantasies, only to ratchet up our own emotional response," Sloane said.

Instead, they looked at Steve's health with a practical eye. "Things could have been bad," Sloane said. "But wasn't it great that they weren't? For some reason, Steve recognized the signs, and we got [to the hospital]. We are really grateful."

Steve's strength also comes from a personal philosophy about death: "My way of thinking is, you won't know it [when you die]. I accept that. You'll just go to sleep, and you won't wake up. But you won't know that you didn't wake up." That's why Steve doesn't think there is anything to worry about.

"I assume I'll wake up," he said. "And if I do, I have a day before me, and a number of things to do."

Chapter 3:   Erin Peiffer

Erin Peiffer didn't want to be awake. Many patients prefer to watch the procedure on the screen: some find it interesting, others want to see with their own eyes if a blockage exists.

Not Erin. Bad news can always wait. The thirty-nine-year-old working mother of three from Eldersburg, Maryland, dozed off while the wire with a balloon attached at the end entered her blood vessels in search of a problem.

Erin had been admitted to Johns Hopkins Hospital in Baltimore, one of the best medical facilities in the country, because her stress test had shown a "blip." That's what the doctor had called it. He didn't think it was much—at least that's what he told his patient—but just to be sure, just to rule out the rare possibility that a woman Erin's age had a blockage, he ordered an angiogram. It was the beginning of some spiraling events that would forever change her life and the lives of her husband and children. Cardiovascular disease can do that.

Erin was groggy from the sedative, but there were so many people in the room when she awoke that she was immediately concerned. Bryan was crying, too emotional to talk because his wife was going to die unless doctors moved quickly.

*   *   *

Erin O'Connell Peiffer had been raised in the middle-class town of Ellicott City, Maryland. That's where she got her first dose of really bad news, the kind that immediately changes your life and the lives of those around you: When Erin was only sixteen, her father, an oral surgeon and an officer in the Naval Reserve, died in an automobile accident, leaving his wife, Beverly, to finish raising the family.

"I don't know how to put it all into words," Erin said of her father's death. "My youngest brother was six, and there were six kids, and my mom hadn't been in the workforce for eighteen years."

Somehow, the family made due, although money was initially a concern for Erin's mother, who openly feared she might eventually need to send the children to live with relatives. It turned out, however, that Erin's father had established a trust fund for the family. It wasn't much, but it was enough to help them get by.

Erin's mother kept her children and even managed to send them to college." She did a damn good job," Erin said. "I tell her now, 'As an adult with half as many kids as you had, I don't know how you did it.'"

Erin earned a degree in social work from Western Maryland College (which isn't really in the western part of the state), and after college went to work helping disadvantaged people. "I was going to save the world. I had all these idealistic views," she said. The idealism included some naiveté about how much money she would need to live comfortably. "I remember thinking when I first got out of college in 1983 that if I could just make $30,000, I would be set."

Erin was a Type A personality, driven, at times aggressive, and almost always needing to be in charge. There are too many surprises when important outcomes are left to others, too many disappointments when they fail to meet her expectations. Interestingly, it's a common trait among the heart-attack survivors I profile in this book.

Erin was competitive, and, quite frankly, social work just wasn't cutting it. The work wasn't accountable or quantifiable. Erin had no way of being certain she was making a lasting difference in challenged people's lives.

At about the same time, she was coming to grips with the fact that $30,000 a year wasn't enough to buy the kinds of things she wanted and needed. Erin would later learn to distinguish between the two.

By the mid-1980s she had left her job in social work—and the apartment in Gaithersburg, Maryland, she'd shared with two of her girlfriends from college—and taken a position in the sales division of telecommunications giant MCI outside of Washington. Here, success was measurable. "You knew exactly how you compared to your peers, not only in the office, the county, the state of Maryland, but across the country," Erin said. "I went into a very accountable profession, which brought out my competitiveness, and I did well."

At about the time Erin started at MCI, Bryan Peiffer found himself in Norfolk, Virginia, fresh out of the Navy. Bryan had served in the Atlantic as an electronic technician on the USS *DuPont* and the USS *Vulcan*. Although, a native of Des Moines, Iowa, he came to like the East Coast and decided to settle in the Washington area.

They met when she was twenty-five. Three years later, in 1989, they were married and moved to Eldersburg, not far from where Erin had grown up. It would be an ideal place to raise a family. Their first child, Evan, was born in February 1992. Matthew followed two years later, and Katherine was born in 1996.

Erin Peiffer appeared to have it all. The husband; cute, healthy children; a suburban home; and the "great job." Hers was not the world her mother had inherited. Being a stay-at-home wife or mom was not in Erin's plans.

At MCI she went from an entry-level sales position to a major account representative in two years. She was eventually promoted to global sales. In October 2002, the company sent its top one hundred employees on an all-expenses-paid trip to France. Erin was among them.

In the year Matthew was born, Erin and Bryan bought a four-bedroom, Colonial-style house in an upper-middle-class neighborhood of Eldersburg. "It's middle-class America," Erin said. "We live on a cul-de-sac. There's a recreation field in our back yard. We have a two-car garage, picket fence, and a golden retriever."

"The house isn't a mansion, and it may be [just] a middle-class neighborhood, but it's on the East Coast, where property is expensive."

Erin estimated then that home prices in her neighborhood averaged around $500,000. At the time, Bryan was working at a defense contracting company in Rockville. With two incomes, the couple could afford to send the children to private schools. They took annual vacations and trips to Des Moines so the kids could visit Bryan's parents. Money was never a concern, but as with many families, a health crisis could change that quickly.

"We had a fair amount of disposable income," Bryan said. "We weren't hurting for anything."

When they bought cars, they paid cash. They used credit cards regularly and paid them in full when the statements came. They knew what a lot of couples learn the hard way, that small, unpaid balances skyrocket when only the minimum amount owed is sent in and the credit card company adds on the interest.

"It was a good living and comfortable, and we had savings and retirement plans," Bryan said. "We had everything we needed or wanted." But they worried that their good jobs, and their time commuting to and from work, was having an impact on their children." We were getting our kids up at 5:30 a.m., getting them dressed, feeding them, and rushing around ourselves," Bryan said.

During the day, the children were in daycare. "We'd get home at six o'clock at night, have dinner, and put the kids to bed at seven thirty or a quarter till eight. And what did we have? We could buy just about anything we needed or wanted," Bryan said, "but we didn't have any time with our kids except on the weekends. It was the classic case of somebody else raising our children."

The couple decided that one of them should stop working and stay home with the children. Erin and Bryan discussed it at length—they even consulted a financial adviser. And every way they worked the numbers, they reached the same conclusion: because Erin made the most money, Bryan would quit his job.

At first, Bryan wasn't comfortable with the idea. A lot of men might have balked at the notion of the wife bringing home the bacon while he took care of the kids. "Initially, I didn't see that as the best option," he said. "Financially it made sense, but I wasn't prepared for it."

That wasn't his only hang-up.

"She is a better nurturer than I."

Despite his reluctance, there was no other option. If one of them was to stay home with the kids, it needed to be Bryan. He agreed to try it for a year. Gradually, he adjusted. Life continued to be good.

Until Thursday, February 1, 2001.

"It seemed like a normal, routine Thursday night," Bryan said. "Once every few weeks I was off with the boys, and she did something with our daughter." It was on a Thursday that Bryan was with the boys at Cub Scouts, and Erin was with Katherine, now four, at the pool where Erin had a water-aerobics class.

"If you sit here and are good while Mommy and Nancy dance around with the old ladies," she told Katherine, "I'll take you to the kiddie pool."

About halfway through the class, Erin started coughing. It was a strange cough, accompanied by a rattling in her chest. She went to the side of the pool, resting her elbows on the edge. "I thought, 'That's weird,'" Erin explained later. "I thought I had swallowed some water, or maybe it's the chlorine in the pool."

It was neither.

She climbed out of the water and away from the smell of chlorine. It didn't help. Erin was still coughing and beginning to think something was wrong. She grabbed Katherine, who had started crying over not going to the kiddie pool, and headed home.

Bryan's cell phone rang just before eight that night, just minutes before the Cub Scout meeting was to adjourn. It was Erin.

"I told him he might want to come home right now."

She didn't give Bryan any more information, but her tone concerned him. "It wasn't normal for her to say anything like that or to be that rushed," he said. "So I grabbed the boys and took off for home."

Erin, now home, was having trouble breathing. She was coughing up pink, frothy fluid. "It was blood-stained," she said. She phoned her primary-care physician, who suggested that she go to the emergency room. Bryan got home before she could decide whether to drive herself or wait for him. When he arrived, Bryan wanted to drive her to the emergency room at Carroll County Hospital, about twenty minutes away. But Erin refused. "'No, no,' I told him. 'You stay with the kids. I don't want to upset them. I'll be fine.'"

Always the one in charge, Erin drove herself to the hospital. She was more annoyed than concerned. "I was like, 'Damn, I really can't breathe. And I can't get this coughing to stop.'" The possibility that her heart was part of the problem didn't occur to her. Why would it?

Most women believe breast cancer is their biggest health threat. That's where a lot of the media attention has been for years. Women have been taught that it's older men who should be worried about heart attacks and strokes, right? Wrong.

"If I had thought this was my heart, I would not have driven myself. When I think back on that now, I think, 'Oh, my God. I could have just keeled over right behind the wheel.'"

Erin was immediately admitted into the emergency room. "My vitals must have been whacked, because they immediately took me back. Whatever they read wasn't good."

Things started moving fast; there was a flurry of activity among the doctors and nurses. Erin began to think it might be really serious. But still, she didn't think it was her heart. She was still in her bathing suit when a doctor examined her.

"Your lungs are wet," he said.

"Yeah, duh! I was in the pool," she said. She now laughs at that comment. She thought the pool water had caused her bloody cough.

"That's not what caused it," he shot back.

They gave Erin some medicine and let her rest in an examination room. She still didn't know why she was sick, nor did she ask. But she was feeling better. She was ready to go home to her family. "I thought, 'I'm good to go.'"

Then something curious happened.

"The door opens and a nurse comes in, and she just stops. She looks at me and says, 'Wow, you are too young to be in here.' I said, 'Where am I?' She said, 'You are in the heart room. You are in congestive heart failure and [have] pulmonary edema.'"

Erin was unfamiliar with those terms. "I don't know what that means," she told the nurse, "but it doesn't sound good."

Back at home, Bryan waited for word from his wife. She had been gone nearly three hours. The phone rang at about 11:30 p.m. Finally, it was Erin's voice, and she sounded better.

"I'm feeling a lot better," she said. "They gave me some meds to get rid of the fluid in my lungs." Bryan thought she had just swallowed water.

"Would you like to talk to the cardiologist?" she asked him.

Huh? Bryan didn't know what to say. Why was she being treated by a cardiologist?

"OK."

The cardiologist came on the line. "It's too soon to say that your wife has or has not had a heart attack, but you'd better get up here." Then the doctor hung up the phone.

"That's all he said to me," Bryan said later, fighting tears as he recalled that night. "And I'm like, 'Oh, my God, my wife is having a heart attack.'"

Erin was surprised to learn that it was her heart that was causing her bloody cough. After all, this didn't feel like a heart attack. There was no pain in her chest, arm, or back.

The cardiologist suspected from the beginning that Erin's bloody cough was heart and lung related. His diagnosis, which was immediately shared with the staff, was congestive heart failure and pulmonary edema. Pulmonary edema is a buildup of fluid in the lungs. Congestive heart failure is a condition in which the heart isn't pumping enough blood to the organs.

Even with the diagnosis, Erin wasn't convinced it could be all that serious. She was a young thirty-nine and had only smoked for a brief period in college. She knew of no family history of heart disease. She had gained some weight since college, about thirty pounds, but she wasn't in bad physical shape. Her exercise program once included biking and aerobics classes. She still occasionally exercised, though admittedly much less now.

"I thought chasing three youngsters around and working full-time gave me enough exercise. But I was fooling myself. I wasn't getting any regular aerobic exercise."

Erin did have high cholesterol, which she got from her mother's side of the family. She was diagnosed with it in the 1980s. "My liver kicks out way too much cholesterol," she explained. "It just builds up." Her primary-care physician, however, never recommended a statin or a low-dose aspirin to deal with the problem.

Because heart disease in women had only recently been recognized as a widespread problem, Erin had never been concerned. Apparently, neither had her physicians.

"They didn't really look for things like that," Bryan said. "The doctors were like, 'You're young. You're a woman. You're OK.'"

It turns out that over the years, the arteries around Erin's heart were narrowing. It was the aerobics class in the pool that night that finally set things off.

"Ultimately, that class saved my life," she said. "Because I had so overly exerted my heart, I had a dramatic presentation of something that was seriously wrong. I could have died that night. My heart failure was so bad that fluid was backing up in my lungs, which is why this pink frothy stuff was coming up."

Though her condition was serious, the ER doctor wasn't convinced Erin had suffered a heart attack. There were two possibilities for why she was sick, he said. The most likely cause was a virus that attacked her heart. Less likely, he told her, was that Erin had a blockage.

"You don't fit the risk factors for that," he reassured her.

By the time Bryan arrived at the hospital, there wasn't much going on. Erin felt better, and the cardiologist had left. The hospital staff told Bryan, "Go home. Be with your family." He refused and insisted on staying overnight to be with his wife.

The next morning, Bryan returned home to get the children off to school. He later went back to the hospital to discover that Erin was being discharged. The cardiologist instructed Erin to take off work for two weeks. That would be enough time for her to recover from the virus, which the doctor still suspected was the culprit. He also gave her some medicine—a diuretic or a beta blocker, Erin can't remember which—so her heart wouldn't have to work so hard. Just to be sure Erin's problem wasn't more serious, the doctor wanted her to visit his office in two weeks for a stress test.

"I was kinda shocked that she was coming home," Bryan said. "She was tired and weak."

Erin still wasn't concerned, and on Monday she returned to work. But she still wasn't feeling great. "My heart was definitely different after that event," she said. "It was more agitated, it was rapid."

Looking back, Erin thinks she may have been in denial. "Part of me was really nervous, and part of me didn't want to deal with it. I just thought, 'I'm fine. I just swallowed water, or something funky happened that night. It's not going to happen again.' I thought it was some weird anomaly."

A week or so later, Erin had the stress test. The results *almost* looked normal. There was a "blip" on the results, the doctor said, and if he hadn't seen Erin that night in the hospital, he likely wouldn't have made anything of it. "That's key," Erin said of the cardiologist's decision to investigate further. "Had I gone to a different doctor who had not seen me in the ER, they could have said, 'See yah! You're fine.'"

The cardiologist suggested an angiogram, to look for blockages in her arteries. Erin got a second opinion from a cardiologist at Johns Hopkins. "Yeah," the other cardiologist said, "an angiogram is the next logical step."

Erin had the procedure done at Johns Hopkins a month after her emergency room visit. She continued to reject all the evidence that pointed to her heart. "As we were driving to Hopkins, I kept telling Bryan to turn around, that this was unnecessary," she said.

Bryan remembers that too: "She was insisting she was fine, and that there was no problem, and that they didn't need to do this." To underscore her point, Erin stubbornly walked five flights of stairs to the angiogram room at Hopkins.

"In hindsight," Bryan said, "having the results of the angiogram that day, she was lucky to have made it to the fifth floor."

During the procedure, Bryan sat or paced in the waiting room. It seemed to be taking too long. He was worried. "I kind of had an idea that things weren't good when I was sitting in the waiting room for quite a while." The room was full, and Bryan could see what happened when doctors delivered good news. "I'd see nurses or doctors come in and say, 'Things went well,' or, 'We put a stent it.'"

When Erin's doctor finally appeared, all he said was, "Can I see you my office?" That was a bad sign.

Erin had a severe blockage, the doctor said, and it was located at a "Y" in her artery. It was too big an impediment to be cleared with angioplasty and a stent.

Meanwhile, Erin awoke from the angiogram to a crowded room. Here's how she describes it:

"When I woke up the room was full of people, including my husband. And he was crying. So, I am like, 'What's going on.' He was too emotional to talk. Then the doctor knelt down and said, 'Erin, you need surgery, and you need it now. You have a 99 percent blockage in your left main—

the big one, the widow maker. Or widower maker, in your case.' And he said, 'If you don't have this done, you have a less than 1 percent chance of being here in four months. You will just drop dead of a massive heart attack.'"

Erin didn't have time to think. Not enough time to get angry, not even enough time to get scared. Her heart surgery had to be done immediately, as quickly as they could gather the surgical team. She didn't hesitate.

"OK. Sign me up. Let's do it."

Things started moving fast. "In hindsight," Erin said, "it was probably best that I had no time to think about what was about to occur, because I would have been petrified." A surgical team was mustered for a double bypass first thing the next morning.

That night Bryan went home to be with the children and tell them their mommy was sick. "I told them that the doctors had to operate on her to fix things. . . . I told them it was her heart, and that they would be able to fix it. And that when she got home she would be in a lot of pain, so they would have to take it easy on her."

The children had mixed reactions, and Bryan didn't know if they understood or if he was just scaring them. All they really understood was that Mommy wasn't coming home right away.

Bryan went back to the hospital to be with Erin the night before the surgery. The hospital staff came for her early the next morning.

"There was a point that my husband had to leave," she said. "They call it 'the kiss-and-go.' . . . I was petrified that I wouldn't make it, and I started to cry. And Bryan said, 'Honey, you gotta go.' Then they put in the IV, and I was out."

Coronary artery bypass surgery is a relatively common procedure. Think of it as a traffic detour: the artery is the highway, the clog a traffic jam. Doctors, in effect, create the detour, allowing traffic to flow around, rather than through, the clog. They open the patient's chest and reroute blood around clogs using healthy arteries or veins taken from the patient's legs or chest. Erin's doctors used arteries from her chest—her internal mammary glands.

Erin's bypass was successful, and she was home after six days. Initially she was helpless, stuck in bed or in a chair, unable to be the mother and wife she once was. It was hard to be in charge when she was often on her back. "Bryan pretty much ran this household," Erin said. "He took the kids to school, he made the meals . . . he would come up and bring me a tray with my breakfast."

He also came home to make Erin lunch and to bring her anything she needed. "He did everything," she said.

Things were made a bit easier with the help of family and friends. "We had a phenomenal support system from the neighborhood and my family," Erin said. "Meals were brought here. They came over to clean. It was a very humbling experience."

And it was emotionally hard for Erin. "[It was] very difficult not to be able to help; very difficult to watch him struggle," Erin said. "And I felt guilty for all the stress I put him under."

Three weeks after surgery, Erin developed Dressler's syndrome, a complication in which the sac around the heart, known as the pericardium, becomes inflamed and filled with fluid. The lungs can fill, too. The condition is thought to be caused by the response of the immune system to the damaged heart. Dressler's used to be more common, affecting 3 to 4 percent of heart-attack survivors. But because of medical advances, it's now extremely rare. According to Erin, only four in one hundred thousand heart patients develop it.

Erin was one of those four.

"My heart got fluid around it, and so did my lungs. I felt terrible. I couldn't lie down flat; I was sleeping in a La-Z-Boy chair, and it hurt like crazy." She also had a fever and wasn't breathing well.

Erin was hospitalized again and given medication for the fluid around her heart. But there was too much fluid around her lungs—they would need to be drained manually.

Six weeks after surgery, Erin started cardiac rehab. Like so many other young heart-attack victims, she couldn't fit in: the other patients were a lot older, feeble, and resigned to their fate. "I hated it. HATED IT," she said. "It was all old folks, and I was the only woman. It was like switching schools in the middle of the year, and when you walk in, everyone stops to look at you."

The experience was made worse by the nurse's reaction on the first day. "I think you are in the wrong place," she said to Erin, not expecting a young woman.

"Honestly, I wish I were," Erin replied.

There were more medical complications. Erin started having terrible pain where her doctors had cut her open for the bypass surgery. As with most other bypass patients, the doctors closed her chest with wire clips. But her doctors used about twenty clips, more than is normal. They did so because when both mammary arteries are used for the bypass, there is a greater chance the chest won't heal well. Erin's clips kept popping and clicking, and were terribly painful. She went back to the hospital to have them removed.

There were other complications, some from the surgery, some from medication. "As often as not, over the course of the next year she was in the hospital with one thing or another," Bryan said. Erin added, "Everything felt like it was crashing down." She estimates she was in the hospital a dozen times in the first year.

The Family and Medical Leave Act allows employees to take up to twelve weeks off from work for certain medical conditions. During this period, employees retain health benefits and are ensured that their jobs will be available when they return. Medical leave, however, is unpaid. For much of the winter, spring, and summer of 2001, Erin was out of work, and the family had no income. The once-financially secure couple was seeing their best-laid plans fall apart: their nest egg was nearly empty. Bryan would have to start looking for a job.

"The idea was that I would take over," Bryan said.

In June, he started sending out resumes. There were a few hits and a few interviews in the summer, but no job offers. Then, on Sept. 11, terrorists flew hijacked commercial planes into the Twin Towers of the World Trade Center in New York.

"The job market completely froze up," Bryan said. He had no leads for some time afterward. Bryan still feels regret over not finding work faster. "I know she wasn't real happy that I didn't find work very quickly. In hindsight, maybe I wasn't looking hard enough."

Erin was recovering, though she was nowhere near healthy. "I was still having issues. I was dehydrated and passing out. They were adjusting a lot of my meds." But by the end of summer, her medical leave was gone. She had to go back to MCI to keep her job. Erin reported back for full-time work that September. She had no other choice: there were no jobs for Bryan, and her family had to eat.

"She was working and not healthy, and I wasn't [working] and was healthy," Bryan said. He felt sick about the situation. "That was tough on her and tough on me, too, because I didn't feel like I was helping her out or doing enough."

Erin worked through the holidays. In January she became very sick and was admitted to Johns Hopkins with an arrhythmia. Then she received a letter from MCI telling her she had used up all her leave time, and if she wasn't back at work in two days, she'd lose her job.

Erin phoned MCI's human resources department from her hospital bed. "Look at your caller ID," she screamed into the phone to the HR rep. "I'm not at the beach."

It didn't matter. The Family and Medical Leave Act measures time off within a twelve-month period, not a calendar year. "You should have waited another month to get sick," someone at human resources told her. "We are sorry. It's already in the HR logs."

Erin couldn't make it back to work in time, and now she and Bryan were both unemployed.

The bad news would not let up. Most of Erin and Bryan's savings, $500,000, had been in her company-issued MCI stock. At the same time she was getting sick, telecom stocks began to tank. In July 2002, MCI WorldCom filed for bankruptcy. News reports said company officers had used fraudulent accounting to boost the firm's stock price. Bernard Ebbers, MCI's founder and chief executive officer, was sentenced to twenty-five years in prison. The Peiffers' half-million dollars in stock was now worth $69.

"Was I despondent? Yeah. I lost my job. I lost my savings," Erin said.

"[It felt like] everything she had worked so hard for wasn't going to be there," Bryan said.

The job market eventually improved. In 2002, Bryan was able to find work as a buyer at a nuclear-waste remediation company in Columbia, Maryland. It was a good job, but Bryan's salary didn't match what his wife had been earning. Erin had been off work long enough to qualify for medical disability payments from Social Security and MCI's insurance carrier. It obviously helped with the family bills, but it was well below her MCI salary.

Then, without warning, Bryan was laid off his job when his company lost a contract. Before, the family's biggest concern was Erin. Would she make it through the surgery? Would she recover? What could they do to make it easier on her? Now, in addition to that, there were financial worries. They had built a life around Erin's MCI income—an expensive life, a life with three kids and a mortgage. Now they had medical expenses and no income.

"Financial hardship was probably the biggest change to the family," Bryan said.

"We moved the kids from private school to public school," Erin said. "We watch the dimes. We stretch. Vacations are few and far between."

At one point, Bryan and Erin were unsure if they could keep the house, because they couldn't pay the mortgage. Plus, the house was financed with an adjustable rate mortgage, and the seven-year fixed period was ending; the rate was about to rise. "We weren't sure, with her health, if we could refinance," Bryan said.

They didn't lose their home, but the bills were piling up all around them, including credit-card debt—something they swore they would never let happen. The trips to Des Moines and the once-a-year vacations stopped—traveling had become too expensive. "We don't get out there very often," Bryan said. "It's sad, because the kids don't get to see their grandparents but once every couple of years. And the grandparents don't get to see their grandkids."

Erin's medical bills were a constant worry and a strain on the family's finances. For a while there was COBRA, a law that lets former employees retain their health benefits for limited periods. But COBRA is expensive, especially considering that those on it usually aren't working. Erin and Bryan were paying more than a thousand dollars per month. On top of that there were the copays. They couldn't afford the coverage, but they couldn't afford to be caught without health insurance. Then someone found a solution.

The trust fund Erin's father had established before he died years earlier included a clause allowing withdrawals for medical expenses. "My mom got permission," Erin said. "We took out the exact amount we needed."

Not surprisingly, Erin was often depressed. She worried about her children and husband, but more than anything else, she wanted to know how much time she had left to be with them. Having heart disease at age thirty-nine doesn't bode well for a long life, she thought. Over and over, Erin drilled her cardiologist: "How long do I have to live?" But the doctor just turned the question back on Erin. "How would you live differently?" she'd ask.

"I would stop worry about saving for retirement and have a really good time," Erin replied. Still no answer from the doctor. "She was the queen of tap-dancing," Erin said.

Then Erin rephrased the question. "Do I have the same life expectancy as my peers?"

At last she got an answer. "No."

How could I not have known I was so sick? Erin would later ask. Was I not paying attention to my body? Is it my fault?

Erin was determined never to be caught unaware again. She became almost fanatical about her health. She got thin, near anorexic. "I went overboard. I was fanatical, certain another shoe was going to drop." If she died, Erin didn't want her children to think she had given up. "I wanted them to see that Mommy really did try."

Bryan could see her fear. "For a while she was hyper vigilant about everything. She was concerned about not seeing her children grow up." One day, Bryan told Erin, "You are living to die." The children had been affected, especially Katherine.

"After the surgery, she would not leave my side," Erin said. "When I went to my very first checkup, she said to me, 'Please don't go Mommy. They are going to keep you again. The last time you went to the doctor you disappeared for a week.'"

It took awhile for the children to adjust, but they did, eventually becoming used to their mommy being away in the hospital.

It was hard on Bryan, too. There was the real possibility he'd be left to raise their four-, six- and eight-year-old children by himself. "It was horrible on him," Erin said. "If the roles were reversed, I don't know if I could have held up as well as him."

Bryan is pragmatic about it, saying he just did what needed to be done. Once, Erin asked him if he'd ever considered leaving her. "Yeah," he replied, "but I want to take you and the family with me. I want to run away from all *this*."

*   *   *

What's still hard is the unpredictability of heart disease. "It's hard to plan stuff," Erin said. "We can plan to go with the kids to Hershey Park on Saturday, and then I get out of bed and I'll say, 'Mommy can't go.'"

"Part of the problem for me is getting used to the fact that this is a forever thing. It's not just, 'Do this for six months and you will be good to go.' It is truly an entire lifestyle."

Now Erin is more realistic about her health. She walks three miles a day (even though she hates it), and she eats well. She looks healthy, vibrant. Time has taught her there is a difference between admitting illness and accepting it. Acceptance brings surrender, and surrender can be the beginning of healing.

The experience has also caused Erin to change her outlook on life, to realize what's important. Before, it was her career that drove her. "I was racing along, racing for money, climbing, and working my way up the pecking order. My self-worth was how much money I made. I was into that groove and all the trappings. Suddenly, with heart disease, the money and material things didn't matter. The most important thing is the connection that you have with other people, family and friends."

Erin can't say enough good things about Bryan. "He is warm, loving, generous and sensitive; an incredible father and wonderful husband. I am very, very fortunate."

Erin won't ever be well enough to return to work. Bryan now has a job as an operations planner at a company that builds unmanned surveillance blimps called aerostats. The family has health insurance through his company, but that plan doesn't pay much for medication. Fortunately, Erin also has coverage under Medicare.

Erin spends much of her time these days passing on what she has learned to others. It's become her passion to make others aware of female heart disease, to bring it out of the dark. Others, she feels, must know that heart disease is the No. 1 killer of women.

"It's a club that you don't want to belong to, and one that I want to keep other women out of," Erin said. "We need to educate the doctors. If a skinny white chick walks in your office complaining of chest pain, don't blow it off. If it was a male, you'd have him doing a cardiac test."

But women must also be educated to take the symptoms of heart attack seriously. "As women, being caretakers, we tend to put ourselves last," Erin said. "We make excuses—ignore symptoms."

Chapter 4:   Hurst Bousegard

Hurricane Katrina tore through New Orleans in August 2005, and "The Big Easy" was left gasping after levees built to protect the city were punctured. What followed was the biggest evacuation in U.S. history

Hurst Bousegard was among the angry people forced to flee and then watch from a distance as his once-vibrant hometown was swallowed up by the Gulf of Mexico. Hurst had spent much of his adult life on the water. At age 48, the seaman, was already a likely candidate for coronary disease, maybe even a heart attack. The country's No. 1 fatal disease had already claimed his grandfather and his dad, Big Hurst.

The stress from Katrina was enough to bring on a cardiac event. Thousands of people were herded into the Superdome, hidden under overpasses, thrown into filthy waters. Bodies were passed over in the streets. Hospital emergency rooms were closed, and families lost touch with loved ones.

It was a Saturday morning when Mayor Ray Nagin appeared on live television calling for a voluntary evacuation of New Orleans. Hurst didn't waste time.

"At 10 a.m., I sprang into action to get the hell out of town to beat the crowd," he said. "I packed up the majority of my clothing, valuables, and laptop, and I was on the road heading west toward Houston."

Later that afternoon, Nagin was on radio and television issuing a mandatory evacuation order for the entire city.

Hurst knew what hurricanes were capable of, and his mind was racing with thoughts of the wind sending the large oak tree branches near his duplex through the roof. He had been born in New Orleans, but Bayou Lafourche, a rural community, some miles to the south, is where he and his siblings grew up.

"It had always been my childhood dream to live in the city of New Orleans—a city with so much soul and personality that just a day visit was like a vacation," Hurst said. "Bayou Lafourche was rural, so many times the citizens of Bayou Lafourche would travel to the city for major purchases and services—especially medical ones, like birthing babies and getting operations; hence, my birthplace. My dream became reality when I received a phone call in early 2000 from one of my close friends, Perry Martin, who was living in New Orleans and looking for a roommate to share expenses. I paid him a visit to check out the area, the apartment and discuss terms. All was agreeable, and I soon became a New Orleans resident in the Mid-City area, centrally located between the French Quarter and City Park. My off-time in New Orleans fueled a party lifestyle, and all was great."

After fleeing Katrina, Hurst landed at his brother Wess' house in Montgomery, Texas, 40 miles north of Houston. "I figured I'd spend the weekend with him until the storm blew through and return home in a few days, which had always been the normal procedure in the past."

Everyone soon learned that Katrina was anything but ordinary. The first television reports said there was wind damage. New Orleans appeared to have dodged a direct hit when Katrina moved more to the east and struck the Pearl River, toward the Louisiana-Mississippi line.

Then the unthinkable happened—something the weather forecasters could not have predicted, a phenomenon for which the Army Corp of Engineers had never prepared the citizens.

"I'm watching with open-mouthed dismay as the TV cameras are showing broken levees with the water pouring into the city," Hurst said. "'Oh, my God,' I said to myself. 'New Orleans is getting destroyed.' As long as I've been around New Orleans, which was most of my life, I never knew that the city was basically 'a bowl surrounded by soup.' I only knew that some parts were below sea level, not the whole thing!"

Hurst was convinced he had lost everything. "I was heartbroken and just plain pissed off." Little did he know that inside his chest there really *was* a broken heart that was about to give out. Hurst would ignore the symptoms—the warnings—until it was nearly too late.

With most communication into New Orleans cut off, it took a week to get a call from his roommate. Perry was OK, and despite his earlier bravado had decided to leave their house at the last minute. Hurst, in Texas, remained glued to the television images. There were reports the government was reacting too slowly, or not at all. "Looters were out of control," Hurst said. "Gangs were actually shooting at rescue helicopters. I got really angry and decided never to live in New Orleans again."

The flood damage was beyond anyone's imagination. "And to think, New Orleans and the Bayou Lafourche area was on the west side of the storm, which is the *good* side to be on. The irony was incomprehensible and unacceptable."

It took a couple of weeks for Hurst to find out that all his family members had fared well, but the condition of his rented duplex apartment, which was in the middle of "flood central," was still a mystery.

It turned out the water missed entering their place by four inches, but the rest of the neighborhood was in ruins. The roommates filled a U-Haul and spent the night in Bayou Lafourche at the home of another friend, Kirk. Bayou Lafourche had electricity, while much of New Orleans was still in the dark.

Before Katrina, Hurst had begun seeing a cardiologist, partly because he didn't want to be caught off guard like his father and grandfather, but mainly to get his sister Angelique off his back.

The grandfather they never knew died at thirty-five. High blood pressure was the stated cause. Hurst was there when his own dad passed away after practically inviting a heart attack to come get him.

Big Hurst had started smoking cigarettes, heavily, around age fourteen or fifteen. Hurst Junior recalled that "due to his heavy smoking, family history and lack of physical activity, he suffered his first massive heart attack at the age of thirty-five, in 1974. He continued to smoke, three to four packs daily, eating anything he wanted and rarely leaving his bed, now using his condition as an excuse. He was also diagnosed as a diabetic. Over the next fourteen years, he would suffer a few more attacks, and he eventually reached a point to where the doctors told him he would not survive another one. He finally succumbed to cardiac arrest at home at age forty-nine. My brother Casey and I were there when he died."

Hurst swore many times prior to Katrina that he wasn't going out the way his old man did. He felt Big Hurst had simply quit on life. Hurst tried without much success to cut back on his own cigarette habit of at least a pack a day. He tried to control his drinking. And there was that promise to his sister, a cardiac nurse, that he would get an annual physical and follow the doctor's advice.

But then Katrina hit and knocked Hurst off his program.

"It was destruction by water instead of bombs," he said. "The air was so putrid with the stench of rotted food in everyone's refrigerators and freezers that there weren't even any birds around—no chirping, none flying about, no moving vehicles. The city was dead still and quiet, except for an occasional other vehicle driving around, which were very few. It was a definite '10' on the eeriness scale. There were mountains of trash everywhere."

The stress alone would have been excuse enough to continue smoking and drinking. Like his neighbors, Hurst was made a nomad by Katrina. A healthy heart wasn't even on his mind. People were worried about where they would live, eat and work.

Hurst had been trying to start an online business when the hurricane hit. Afterward he tried to jump-start the enterprise, but with little success. Most of his belongings were stuffed in a storage facility somewhere. He kept just the basics with him at his brother's house in Texas.

"There was some temporary emergency money from FEMA and the Red Cross but that didn't last long."

Four months after the storm, in January 2006, Hurst had to make a big decision. It had nothing to do with his health, but everything to do with where he would live and how he would make a living.

"I relocated back to Bayou Lafourche temporarily to finish out the jewelry business for the Mardi Gras season and then get a job working on another boat. I stayed with Kirk for a while and rented his mother's spare efficiency apartment, fully intending to move permanently to Texas near Wess, where the elevation is 246 feet *above* sea level. No more flooding for me. I just needed a new job to settle into and research the area north of Houston where I might relocate."

When all else failed—and it did—Hurst knew he would go back to sea. One of the benefits of being a sailor is that you can always find work and live virtually anywhere. He easily landed a job with Delta Towing Company in Houma, Louisiana. The money was good, at times great. There was always a shortage of skilled boatmen, meaning Hurst could work as many hours as he wanted. "The most money and benefits I ever had," He said.

He found a new roommate, John, who also worked with Delta Towing. "John and I got along well because we had some things in common—we were educated, avid readers." Hurst had three years of college and preferred nonfiction, biographies, and crime stories.

"John and I were well-mannered, easy-going guys, similar sense of humor, and we were both addicts to nicotine and wanted to quit. John was a newlywed with a nonsmoking wife, so she was putting the pressure on him, and I've been trying to quit totally since the day I started thirty years ago. I made many attempts but would always eventually fall off the wagon."

They were sailors working on an offshore tugboat that moved oil rigs from location to location in the gulf, wherever needed, for drilling operations.

Hurricanes Katrina and then Rita caused catastrophic damage to the offshore oil industry; at the same time the demand for oil was climbing because of booming economies in China and India. This kept Hurst and John at sea, away for weeks on end from the mainland, where the good doctors and regular checkups could be found.

Boat companies made it seem worth their while. Captains and mates easily earned six-figure salaries. The only requirement was some experience and a license from the Coast Guard.

"You didn't even need a high school diploma," Hurst said. "My friend John has a college degree in psychology; but was working as a deckhand on the boat and making nearly *twice* the money he could have commanded as a social worker or counselor."

Hurst had carved out a niche on the tugboat as a cook. "I was making more money on the boat as a cook than I ever have in my life, and was happy as a blue collar. You could actually see the results of your work, every day was different, our operations were totally spontaneous, and my cooking skills were sufficient enough to put smiles on most of my crewmates' and captains' faces."

Hurst enjoyed being in control of his time. Katrina had taken that away. "I decided how long to stay on the boat, when to go home, and when to return to the boat. My money was my own, and I was able to live the lifestyle I dreamed about." He described his life then as a series of two-week vacations.

"There was ten days in Tahiti for my fortieth birthday. I explored Mexico for three weeks. Later, a ten-day jaunt along the California coast with a rented red convertible. There were trips in the Bahamas; a week in Puerto Vallarta, Mexico; a couple of Amtrak trips across the country."

He'd never consider that lifestyle reckless or purely self-centered. But Hurst admitted there were lots of women, shameless sexual activity, boozing, and all-night partying, often with people he hardly knew or cared to know for long.

"Being a single, independent man afforded me the luxury of traveling alone, which I enjoyed, because it provided total freedom. There was no one else to answer to, and I was able to do anything I wanted at any time, whether kicking back to relax or being the party animal. Besides, any desire for female companionship could be accomplished at my destinations."

"I once read a silly statistic that women are fourteen thousand times more likely to engage in casual sex while on vacation *even if their husbands are present.* My experiences proved this to be true, most of the time; but I would stay away from the married ones. I just happened to have a limit to my debauchery."

Was he trying to fit a lifetime into but a few years, knowing how little time his father and grandfather had been given?

"I enjoyed drinking, but it was never a real problem except when I was drunk enough to be sick the next day. I can take it or leave it— alcohol was never addictive for me. Living the offshore life was a matter of extremes. When you go to work, you disappear from home for a month, and when you return home, you're home for two weeks straight. Therefore, whenever a sailor gets home, he's got some 'catching up' to do with all aspects of life's pleasures. My two big pleasures other than the Internet dating scene were gambling and drinking, besides the smoking.

They sort of worked hand in hand, so when I went gambling, I would naturally drink, and I was doing too much of both."

Hurst began to experience blackouts. He'd wake up some days late and not knowing what he did the night before or how he got home. He would check his wallet for receipts, cash withdrawals, and look outside to see if his car was there and undamaged.

Recovering alcoholics would say Hurst was ripe for an intervention.

He rationalizes that, "Everything checked out OK each and every time, except for the fact that I was blowing a lot of money at the casinos. I got the drinking under control by slowly sipping red wine instead of hitting the rum and Cokes."

Hurst admits he was a compulsive gambler, but whether it was a real problem is a matter of opinion. "The only money I was losing was discretionary income. I always made sure my bills were paid on time, I had an excellent credit rating, and I was maxing out my 401(k) contributions at work, so the only money I was throwing away was money I could have saved or made additional investments."

Hurst stopped reminding himself that he probably had a date with destiny. He hadn't seen his cardiologist in more than two years. People with no fixed address usually don't bother.

"Part of my Katrina relocation plan was to see my doctor before leaving for Texas, informing him of my situation but staying on as his patient so I could get my annual workup whenever I'd get off the boat. But first I needed to call his office to see if he was still in town. Katrina had chased off many medical professionals due to the closing of most of the hospitals. As the old saying goes, 'So much for well-laid plans.'"

Then it hit him. One day as Hurst and John were traveling to work on the tugboat, he began getting a funny feeling in the middle of his chest. "It started off like heartburn, but then settled into a tiny sharp pain in the center of my chest. Whenever I would take a deep breath, I felt soreness near the bottom of my lungs."

He didn't for a minute consider it might be heart related. "My knowledge of heart disease had not led me to believe that it was cardiac related because the pain was not throbbing, nor was it that bad. My suspicion was emphysema."

"As I drove along, the funny feeling would get worse, and then lessen. This went on for about twenty minutes, and I came very close to having John drop me off at a hospital." But in Hurst's mind, there were a lot of reasons not to head to the hospital. "That would have messed up my work schedule, provide major inconvenience to other captains and the company, delay my move again." He just didn't have time to be sick. Not right now.

He had John pull into a convenience store lot. Hurst went inside and picked up a snack and some aspirin. "I decided to keep quiet about it," he said. "But I also decided to not touch another cigarette, which lay on the seat beside me. It was time to get serious."

Hurst and John eventually reached the boat and went through the usual procedures for unloading their gear before settling into their rooms.

"I noticed that all the activity, especially walking up and down the stairs, winded me more than usual. I decided to give it a few days to see how things developed. My mind raced with all the physical possibilities that could be occurring with me, so I decided not to take any more chances than necessary. I took it as easy as I could without raising suspicion from anyone that something may be wrong."

The plan for the rest of the time he was offshore, a full twenty-eight days, was to take an aspirin every day and not go through his usual exercise routine.

There was another vow to quit smoking. "This time I made it a point to write down in my date book 'Last Cigarette' on Sept. 19. That way, I'd have my quit date recorded and a reason to celebrate a year later. Somehow I knew that no matter what the outcome, there would be no more cigarettes."

A few days later, the small, sharp pain in his chest was still there. "It was like someone had stuck me in the chest ever so slightly with a straight pin and just left it there. The daily aspirin would lessen the pain during the day, but [it] was waiting for me when I awoke each morning."

Hurst eventually made the phone call he had been putting off to his sister. Because she was a registered nurse, her siblings always consulted her before going to the hospital. When Hurst told her about the pain in his chest that had by now been lingering for weeks, her response was quick and without sympathy.

"Gee, Hurst, let's see . . . our father died of heart disease, you're a smoker, and you have chest pain. What do you *think* is happening?"

Hurst continued to procrastinate. "I felt fine, my symptoms didn't feel to be cardiac related, but it was that very small, sharp, annoying pain in my chest that had me concerned. My suspicion was emphysema, and I had no desire to leave the boat unless it was absolutely necessary. It was a personal trait I had—not to inconvenience others unnecessarily, and getting off the boat now would cause a few small wrenches to fly."

His was a classic case of denial.

"Well, it's your call," Angelique said. "But if the pain stays the same, or if it gets any worse, then you need to get off the boat and to an emergency room as soon as possible."

"I promised her I would," Hurst said. He would later discover that what he began experiencing in the vehicle that first day of work was what's known as a silent heart attack—a mild heart attack whose symptoms are often mistaken for something else, like heartburn, indigestion, even emphysema.

"As the days went by, I found my 'condition' improving," Hurst said. "The pain was lessening slowly but surely, and my shortness of breath was disappearing. I started to relax more but kept up the regimen of daily aspirin. As luck would have it, we became short of a deckhand on the boat, which meant I had to fill in whenever we hooked up to a rig to move it. It required heavy lifting, and moving of solid steel equipment. Fortunately, the entire operation only took fifteen to thirty minutes, much of it waiting to make the right moves at the right time. But the activity got me extremely short of breath, and it was noticeable by Captain Kelvin. "What's the matter, old man?" he joked. "Out of shape are we?" I would nod and smile, and eventually got my breath back in about five minutes."

By the middle of the twenty-eight-day tour, Hurst was becoming concerned that maybe, just maybe, the situation could be heart related.

He put in a call to his original cardiologist. His appointment with Dr. Stanley Bleich of East Jefferson Hospital, in the New Orleans suburb of Metairie, was set for Monday, October 22, nearly three years after Katrina had hit.

"I had always enjoyed seeing him and going through all the barrage of tests. First of all, I was always the youngest patient in the waiting room.

Secondly, whenever the doc would finish consulting with his patients, you can hear the exiting conversation from the waiting room. 'See you in three months,' he would tell an elder patient, or, 'See you in six months,' he would tell another. Whenever he would be done with me, he would always say, 'Well, young man, all I can tell you is, see you next year.' Always a clean bill of health, without a trace of blockages or other heart-related maladies."

But that was three years ago. A lot can change in that time for someone with cardiovascular disease.

"I was expecting to hear something a little different this time around. I did the usual nuclear stress test, EKG, and heart ultrasound. The technician for the stress test informed me that everything appeared to be fine, but the doc would have to study it, get back to me, and that I could now go home. I traveled back to my apartment in Bayou Lafourche to kick back and watch television."

Later that night, his cell phone rang. It was Dr. Bleich. Getting a call from a cardiologist at home, at night, following a battery of tests, can be a bit unnerving.

"Looks like you definitely have a blockage, so we need to do an angiogram ASAP. That will tell us how large the blockage is, and if it's 70 percent or greater. Then we'll be able to put in a stent at that time."

"OK," Hurst said, "no problem. When do you want to do it?" It would be Thursday. "I had a dental appointment the next day and joked to myself that if anything major happened, I would at least have clean teeth."

The control addict emerged. He reflected back, planned ahead with projections and outcomes and consequences. It's typical of a lot of the heart-attack survivors I interviewed for this book. Working on an offshore tugboat, Hurst had a lot of time to think. He thought of every scenario concerning his heart and what each outcome would be.

"I thought it would be a diagnosis of emphysema. I would have to quit smoking, but I would still be able to work. Worst-case scenario would be that I have blockages and would need a bypass operation, which these days, you'd be back home in a week, and I'd have some recuperation time off work. Thanks to the great benefits I had from the company, I was well covered for major medical as well as short- and long-term disability in the event I had to go that route.

"If for some reason I would be disabled, the company would continue to pay me 60 percent of my annual income until the age of sixty-five, which would still allow me to live comfortably in my situation. In short, I was not worried, especially since I made it home without having a heart attack, which I never would have suspected in the first place."

Thursday arrived. Hurst checked into the hospital, with Angelique at his side. The plan was to perform the angiogram, inserting a balloon attached to a wire through the groin into an artery. Once the blood vessel is cleared of the blockage, a stent is inserted to keep it open. Hurst would be kept overnight for observation, then sent home the next day.

"I was awake for some of the procedure, which was normal, and was able to see my blockage on the big, flat-screen monitor. It was actually shaped like a portion of the Rocky Mountain range on one side of one of my arteries, and it appeared to be somewhat long. The entire procedure was painless, and I eventually woke up in my hospital room to find Angelique there waiting to let me know the scoop.

"Sure enough, my blockage was 70 percent and required two stents to open that sucker up. The blockage was in the left arterial descending artery, which I would later learn had a nickname by the medical industry: 'the widow maker.' They were keeping me overnight, and I would be home by noon the next day. I was feeling no pain, and obviously they removed the little pin that had been sticking in my chest for nearly a month."

The next morning, Angelique entered his room as preparations were being made to release him. "I would feel a lot better if you stayed overnight at my house at least one more night before going back to the bayou," she said. "That way, if anything unusual develops, you'll be here near the hospital."

It was a Friday, so Hurst assured her he would stay for the weekend, do some partying in the city, and go home Sunday. Angelique had a nice, large home in River Ridge, a suburb of New Orleans, with her husband, Tom, and their daughters Claudia, ten, and Claire, five.

"I was given a prescription for Plavix, which I planned on filling the next morning," Hurst said. "The family usually sleeps in a little on weekends, but I'm stuck being an early riser, so the next morning, a little after 8 a.m., I quietly slipped out of the house to get my prescription filled."

It was October 2007. Hurst would learn that his heart disease would not be cured by one angioplasty and a few stents. His life as a free-spirited tugboat sailor was about to be sunk. A major heart attack was coming—as he drove down Jefferson Highway toward Harahan to fill a prescription at a Wal-Mart pharmacy.

"I start getting sharp jabs of pain dead center of my chest," Hurst said. "No little pinlike discomfort this time. It feels like someone is jabbing me in the chest with an ice pick, and the pain is throbbing and intense. What the hell? I thought—this isn't right! I grab my cell phone to call Angelique, and she answers."

"I told him to hang up and dial 911," Angelique recalled. He didn't listen.

Hurst explained, "I was actually thinking that maybe the stents got crooked, thereby causing the sharp pain, *still* not thinking heart attack." He proceeded to the pharmacy before it became clear that he wasn't going to make it. He pulled off the road for what seemed like a few seconds, just enough time for the pain to subside. Then he put the vehicle in drive again. The pain returned, and this time it was worse. "My breathing hastened, and I began sweating. After about a mile of that, I couldn't take it anymore. I got Angelique back on the phone as I was pulling into the next parking lot, which belonged to the Red White & Blue Thrift Store."

Angelique told him she would meet him there, and that he should call an ambulance.

"911. What is your emergency?"

"Ma'am, I think I may be having a heart attack!"

Hurst was on Jefferson Highway, near the Huey P. Long Bridge. The 911 operator told him to stay on the line until an ambulance arrived. By this time, Hurst was clutching his chest with his left hand, holding the cell phone in his right, and moaning loudly with each stab of pain that occurred with every heartbeat.

A Jefferson Parish police car pulled up. The ambulance arrived seconds later. The paramedics sprang into action, pulling out a gurney. Hurst walked to the stretcher and laid down on it as Angelique arrived.

"I hopped in the back of the ambulance. I knew the paramedics. I had worked with them before," she said.

Hurst was awake and afraid. "This is a heart attack, right?" he asked.

"You are definitely having a cardiac event," Angelique said, having turned into the nurse with a dying patient. "I was behind him, and suddenly he went into V-tach," a potentially life-threatening speedup of the heartbeat. "I was calm, but it was my brother. It's different when it's a family member."

Hurst recalled being in so much pain "my eyes were clenched shut," and he was "still moaning and baying like a hurt animal."

Angelique was prying open his mouth and tossing aspirin down his throat, but still there was no relief. A nitroglycerin tablet under the tongue didn't help either.

Then, Hurst said, "Things began to change. I felt the pain go away and my body relax. No more loud moaning. I felt myself getting sleepy. I thought, 'Thank God, the nitro is working, and the heart attack is ending. Probably a few days in the hospital for observation and all would be well. I was relaxing with my eyes shut, but still awake."

Angelique saw it differently: her patient was dying. "He went into that kind of snore that heart-attack patients get. One of the paramedics said we have to shock him."

Then, *Pow!* Hurst felt an immense electrical shock go through his body.

"My own sister shocked me with those electrical paddles you see on TV when they have to shock someone back to life. It was by far the most jolting pain I've ever felt. It was worse than the heart attack itself."

They arrived at the emergency room of East Jefferson Hospital. Someone removed Hurst's clothes.

"A couple of minutes later, I get shocked again. I screamed. More calm voices, people were reciting numbers, eventually a third shock. I yelled from the pain. More work, more calm voices, more medical gibberish, then a fourth shock and another yell. This time someone actually apologized for shocking me. A male voice said, 'I'm so sorry, sir . . . but we have to do this.' And I actually replied, 'It's OK.' But I was thinking, *Why do they keep shocking me? I thought they only did that to dead people.* That's when the reality of the situation hit me. I kept dying, they kept bringing me back.

"I was not going to die. It simply wasn't my time. I can't explain why I knew it."

The ER team inserted a line into the artery toward the stents. Hurst is sure they hit him again with a defibrillator—in all, seven times.

The next thing he remembers was Angelique coming to his side in the catheterization lab. "They're going to rush you into emergency surgery and give you a triple-bypass operation. Is that OK with you?" she asked.

"There was no hesitation in my voice when I replied, 'You tell them to do whatever it is they need to do. I just don't want to be shocked anymore,'" Hurst told her. "And with that, they began wheeling me away. It was then 9:25 a.m. . . . In exactly one hour, I had survived a massive heart attack followed by seven cardiac arrests."

"My first memory after the operation was waking up to a roomful of family. I asked someone, 'Is it my imagination, or are all my siblings here in the same room at the same time?' It took fifty years to see that happen. I'm talking about people who have never even *met*."

Hurst was the only child from a first marriage. Both his parents remarried and had more children. "I was raised by my mother, Sylvia, and stepfather, Bill Brabits, who produced two sons, Wade and Wess."

Hurst Senior and his wife, Alice, had two daughters and three sons, creating a total of eight half-siblings, with Hurst Junior being the oldest by four years.

"My siblings and I never refer to each other as half-siblings; they are all my brothers and sisters, and I'm close to all of them. My two sisters are both nurses. The oldest, Angelique, is the one who was mainly responsible for saving my life and caring for me afterwards."

"As I would drift in and out of consciousness, I would look up to see who was visiting me that day. My mother and stepfather were there like clockwork every day. They were the ones who had raised me. . . ."

"The combination of the blockage, heart attack, cardiac arrests, the seven shocks, and the bypass surgery gave me heart failure, more specifically, left ventricular, low-output heart failure, which in layman's terms means that the left main chamber of my heart had stopped working *entirely*."

That weakens the heart, which limits the strength of the flow of blood and fluids. When that flow becomes limited, the fluids begin to back up, putting more strain on the vital organs.

Hurst's lungs failed, which meant a respirator would do his breathing. Then his kidneys failed, which meant dialysis would be needed. When Hurst's liver started to fail, the doctor told his relatives they should consider making final arrangements. His seventy-year-old mother wanted to know if her son was dying. "I'm telling you he is *most likely* going to die," was the doctor's response, according to Hurst.

East Jefferson Hospital had no transplant program. Ochsner Medical Center, where Angelique worked, did. It was decided that Hurst wasn't healthy enough to be a candidate. There must have been concern that this sailor might also not have the discipline needed to follow instructions that might one day get him well enough to qualify for a new heart.

Nearly three weeks after his terrifying arrival at East Jefferson Hospital's emergency room, Hurst was transferred to Ochsner Medical Center, where a more aggressive series of treatments was begun. "Within forty-right hours," Hurst said, "my vital organs were functional, and I began the turnaround." It would be a slow recovery.

"I was constantly coughing and having to clutch a pillow to my chest to absorb some of the body's vibration, Hurst said. "I couldn't communicate verbally with anyone and could barely write messages due to my slowed brain function. My scribbling was that of a mentally challenged second grader. I would try using hand signals to no avail. Worst of all, I couldn't sleep. I would sometimes hallucinate and have delusions of paranoia, which is normal for heart patients. I was actually afraid to go to sleep for fear I would not wake up, and I would have sworn on my life that I had not slept in two weeks. The real torture was having a clock on the wall directly in front of me. I would close my eyes for a while, try to sleep, sometimes hallucinate, feel like hours had gone by, and then open my eyes, only to discover that three minutes had passed. I thought of the possibility of actually being in my version of hell, and that's when I started giving up. Why do I have to go through this?"

Hurst had been married and divorced years before in Bayou Lafourche. He had no children.

"I thought, *I have no wife, no kids—no one to leave behind except a bunch of siblings with their own families, a set of elderly parents I only see once or twice a year. What's the big deal? After a week or so of mourning, they'll all continue their lives and go on.* So, one day I wrote the note to Angelique that took up an entire page with large, wriggly letters: 'Why don't you just let me die.'"

It wasn't a question, but a request. Angelique and the rest of the family sprang into full emotional support to change his mind. His oldest sibling told him he could get through this, as did other people. Angelique's thirteen years of nursing gave her credibility when Hurst wasn't willing to trust others, including his own cardiologist. She convinced him the hospital couldn't risk giving a transplant to someone with a chance of developing other serious illnesses like emphysema or cancer. If he smoked, he would be kicked out of the transplant program. If he drank, he could be taken off the transplant list.

The hospital, while boring, was at least safe for the weeks Hurst was there getting his organ functions back. Family members weren't sure he would make it—left to his own demons—once he left Ochsner Medical Center.

Eventually the respirator was removed, the catheter changed. Blood was taken daily. The embarrassment of having the nurses sponge bathe him was long gone. The daily parade of nurses bringing pills and monitoring his IV never let up.

Hurst says he spent those days in a stupor, mentally numb, unable to read, watch TV, or concentrate during conversations that extended past "Yes" or "No" responses. It became painful to even think about his carefree days aboard the tugboat, when every port promised a different type of good time.

Hurst's illness became his family's illness. They were totally absorbed in his condition. It was as though they were saying, "Let us help take care of you and love you until you can learn to do these things for yourself." Eventually Hurst became willing to let them into his space.

"Along with Angelique, there was another person who kept my outlook optimistic on a daily basis. It was my stepdad, Bill. Every single day he was there, Dad would enter my room with notepad and pen in hand to record the readings from my IV monitor. He explained to me what each number represented, and that everyone's main concern was my oxygen saturation and how I needed to breathe more efficiently. He is also, like Angelique, a person who believes that things should be done correctly and effectively, and if something questionable arose, he would get the answers. So when I would see Dad come into my room each day and write those numbers down, I knew he was on top of things and I was going to be fine."

Eventually the transplant team headed by Dr. Hector Ventura concluded that Hurst had become a good candidate for a new heart. He was introduced to two men who had already gotten new organs.

"One had his heart for two years and the other for seventeen years," Hurst said. "They seemed perfectly normal to me and assured me that they were leading normal lives. That was the day my optimism finally stepped up to the plate and I began fighting for recovery in earnest."

"Will I be able to go back to work?" Hurst asked Dr. Ventura, the question every heart patient wants to ask at some point. It wasn't just the job he wondered about; the answer would tell him what kind of life he might expect after his several near-death experiences.

"What do you do for a living?" the doctor asked.

"I work on an offshore tugboat."

The physician grimaced, thought to himself for a few seconds and said, "If you had a desk job, it would have been *possible*. But working offshore? No way."

As the information sank in, Hurst Bousegard was suddenly struck by the realization that he would never work offshore again. He was being retired about fifteen years before his fellow seamen. "I wondered, *What quality life would it be? Will I be able to live on my own again?* As a man, I naturally thought, *Would I ever be able to have sex again?*"

Hurst spent his final three weeks in the hospital with physical therapists. "I was finally standing, showering in a chair, and eventually walking, eating regular food." Hurst had lost forty pounds and looked better than he had in twenty years.

Christmas was approaching, and there was talk that Hurst would be home by Christmas Eve. Angelique and Tom had decided to take him into their home. The only reason Hurst was still in the hospital was to complete intravenous treatment for a staph infection he'd picked up and to receive the IV heart medicine Dobutamine. The hospital wanted him to go to a long-term health-care facility, but Angelique convinced the doctors that she was perfectly capable of handling the situation at home.

Hurst would keep using the IVs at home. They would work by a battery-operated pump, which he'd wear around his waist. His release didn't come until the day after Christmas. Hurst was fully dressed in thick pajamas with his portable pump at his side when Angelique walked into his room and announced, "OK, it's all done. Let's go."

I was confused. I asked, "Aren't they supposed to wheel me out in a wheelchair? Isn't that hospital policy?"

With all the authority she could muster, Angelique said, "Screw that. You're *walking* out of here."

Hurst slowly and gingerly exited the elevator, walked out the hospital exit, and smelled fresh air. "It was a smell I will never forget," he said.

Angelique saw that Hurst was beginning to change. He had been headstrong, impatient. "Riding in a car with my brother [driving] had always been painful. If another driver doesn't brake or use his signal, or stays at the stop sign too long . . ." She didn't finish the sentence. "When we ride together, I drive."

It was raining the day she drove Hurst home from the hospital. Unexpectedly, he started to weep as he gazed out the passenger-side window watching the passing scenery. "I knew that heart patients become more emotional creatures after their experience," Hurst said later, "so now it was my turn."

Angelique noticed and asked, "Are you crying?"

"Yes," he responded, slightly embarrassed. "I'm scared. I'm just really scared. I'm scared of dying."

Angelique explained "Look, first of all, you don't have the type of condition where you can drop dead on my kitchen floor at anytime—I can assure you of that, because if you did, I would not be bringing you to my home and exposing that to my two little girls.

"You have heart failure, which is a slow, degenerative condition. I know what signs to look for, and if you start getting worse it'll be over a period of three or four days. If that happens, all we have to do is get you back to the hospital for more medication, and they'll probably put you on the transplant list at that time. OK?"

It was the first time she explained his condition that way—or was it merely the first time Hurst had listened?

Hurst took up residence at what he called Angelique and Tom's "home-health-care center," and as the weeks and months went by, he began to thrive. He was walking. His muscle tone was coming back, and he was getting up each morning with a new sense of joy.

Some heart patients can become depressed to the point of having suicidal thoughts. Hurst said he never got to that point, but he would sometimes cry for no reason, which he attributed to a chemical imbalance, "much like a woman going through menopause." A change in medication corrected that.

He had a defibrillator/pacemaker implanted on March 12, 2008. "Now I had my own built-in paramedic in case the need arose," he joked.

"I was actually getting healthier despite the weak-heart thing," Hurst said. Doctors discovered that his ejection fraction, which refers to the amount of blood pumped out of a ventricle with each heartbeat, was 20 percent. Anything 40 percent and below puts you in the heart-failure category.

Hurst was told he could lead a normal life as long as he did it slowly and carefully.

His specific condition is called left ventricular heart failure, which means that the left ventricle of his heart is totally nonoperative. The heart is one of the organs that can compensate for weaknesses to a certain extent. But the left ventricle has a direct connection to the respiratory system, so Hurst becomes winded easily.

Sexual intercourse is out. "I would like an intimate relationship," Hurst said. "Only it's hard to find a woman who understands and can deal with my situation."

"Before my heart attack, I never had a problem being alone. It was tranquil and stress-free. However, since the attack, that has changed somewhat. I now get lonely sometimes, but I call up a friend for lunch or dinner, and all is well again. As far as the sexual aspect, my condition has destroyed at least 90 percent of my desire for sexual intercourse, which I do not consider to be a problem—you simply do not miss what you do not desire. But what I *do* miss is simple intimacy with women—that is where my yearning lies. Just to be able to hold someone, kissing and caressing, is what I miss the most, and I would be perfectly content with that alone."

Hurst compares his condition to a vehicle with transmission problems: he can still move down the road and make progress, but only in first gear. And that applies not just to sexual function, but to heart and brain function as well.

Two of the main effects of heart failure are loss of concentration and of short-term memory. "I still cannot read books or magazine articles, because my mind wanders off too much. I can do e-mail fine, but that's about it, so now I'm hooked on audiobooks. And I constantly forget everything within seconds. I have to write down all errands and events in advance—a perpetual 'to-do' list."

Despite all that he has been through, Hurst Bousegard remains a positive person. He says his heart attack, his near-death experiences, and his current physical limitations have made him a better person.

"I do not miss the previous single life—it was, after all, a bit destructive and could have been much worse. The previous life is probably the reason for the heart attack in the first place. My unhealthy desires have been totally destroyed by my cardiac event, and I am very, very thankful for that. It also showed me what the real priorities in life are. I still enjoy traveling, but I am restricted to traveling only to metropolitan areas with major medical centers."

Hurst has a timeshare in Orlando, Florida, outside of Disney World, with a major hospital about the same distance away.

"Since leaving the hospital, I have taken a road trip to Arkansas with two close friends to visit another close friend, road trips to visit relatives, a long weekend in Atlantic City" for some gambling, Hurst said. There's also been a family vacation to Cancun, and a family trip to Kansas City to see a niece graduate from high school.

And there also was another hurricane evacuation—but with far less drama. This time it was Hurricane Gustav, in 2008, and Hurst used the time to visit his parents in Longview, Texas.

"I'm positive almost always. Despite the negative aspects of my condition, I wouldn't trade it for the world. All of my personal relationships have been enriched to a higher level, and it brought two families socially together for the first time in fifty years. I appreciate all the little things the world has to offer—the wind rustling through trees, the warmth of sunshine on the skin, distant barking dogs—things that reflect life in all forms that are overlooked by my fellow neighborhood walkers who choose to plug themselves into their iPods. They don't realize that telling a fellow human 'Hello' does wonders to the soul, and that the natural sounds of a neighborhood could bring peace to the psyche. And of course, a forced early retirement with a comfortable disability income with just enough health to enjoy it doesn't hurt. I realize that not all people are nearly this lucky."

Hurst still lives in the New Orleans area, away from the gulf on higher ground. He lives alone in an apartment and continues to travel and gamble a little. He's no longer waiting for a donor heart. Thus far he has responded well to treatment, and his own big heart continues beating.

"It's shocking," Angelique said. "He is indeed a miracle, and he's now the most compliant patient that I have ever seen."

Chapter 5:   Anita Fox

The priest came into Anita Fox's hospital room in Milwaukee on her second day in intensive care. It was one of those "good news-bad news" situations. If a member of the clergy shows up, it may be a sign that your chances of living a long life may have dropped a bit, yet you want the comfort and assurances that a better existence awaits you on the other side.

Anita was sick, very sick. Just hours before, she had learned she had double pneumonia—and that was after the heart attack. She desperately needed open-heart surgery—her arteries were too clogged for angioplasty or stents—but Anita was far too ill for the operation.

"It was the most overwhelming feeling," Anita explained of that first night in the hospital. "I felt like somebody was trying to smother me with a pillow." It was difficult to process.

That's when the priest appeared in the doorway of her room. He understood that Anita was gravely ill, and he wanted to anoint her. Catholics refer to it as the last rites. In the past, you didn't get this dreaded sacrament, also known as extreme unction, unless you were dying. The church calls it the sacrament of the sick, as discussed in the Book of James: "Is any sick among you? Let him call for the elders of the church, and let them pray over him, anointing him with oil in the name of the Lord. And the prayer of faith shall save the sick, and the Lord shall raise him up; and if he has committed sins, they shall be forgiven him."

Anita was not particularly religious, but she wasn't going to turn the priest away. "I was kinda like, 'OK, I'm not going to say no.'"

At her heaviest, Anita had weighed 270 pounds, and that made it difficult—no, nearly impossible—for her to get around with any comfort. "I did some traveling," she said. "But I couldn't do as much." Once she took a trip to San Francisco. "I had a great deal of trouble with the hills, so I was constantly catching trolleys."

Her weight made exercise and diet seem like "silly ideas." Where to start, and for how long?" she might ask. "I was tired all the time, was just dragging through life." As her weight increased, her self-esteem plummeted. What came first, the excessive weight or the low self-esteem? The chicken or the egg? What difference did it make?

"I was horrified that I felt this way," she said.

Anita saw her primary-care doctor, eager to find out why she had been feeling so sick. She could feel him looking at her and sizing her up. The doctor, she thought, didn't take her symptoms seriously. Fat people's feelings or comments are often not given the weight of thinner, smaller people. It's a fact.

Anita is convinced her doctor figured she was just out of shape, and he was blunt with her. "He essentially looked at me and said, 'Anita, you are fat, you are fifty, and you work too much. What do you expect?'" He sent her home with instructions to lose weight. "No tests," she said of her doctor's diagnosis. "He just palmed it off."

"I went home and cried. It was so callous, so blunt, so insulting." And it wrecked what was left of her self-esteem. "I just figured that I would have to live like that."

Unfortunately, the doctor's response to Anita's symptoms was typical. Many good doctors still don't understand the extent to which heart disease affects women. They often don't know what symptoms to look for in women, because many women have symptoms that appear unrelated to the chest or the heart, such as anxiety, weakness, dizziness, fainting, fatigue, nausea, and shortness of breath. Anita had many of those symptoms.

Doctors lack the high "index of suspicion" necessary when confronted with symptoms that could suggest a looming heart attack in many men and women.

Dr. Elizabeth Ross, a leading cardiologist and author of *Healing the Female Heart*, said that when she was in medical school, there was little information on women and heart attacks. "In the first two weeks after a heart attack, women are twice as likely to die as men" she said. "I think there is a tendency not to refer women for treatment as early. I think there is an assumption in the medical community that women don't get heart attacks, and that women should take care of the men their lives."

The fact is, half of all Americans who die this year of a heart attack will be women, and while breast cancer gets more attention, heart disease causes ten times as many deaths as breast cancer and all other cancers combined. "Women control the heart health of their families. Teach a man and you influence one person; teach a woman and you make a difference to a family," Dr. Ross said.

Anita Fox had no way of knowing her condition could be heart related. She, like her doctor, focused on the obvious problem: her weight. "If I had a clue, I would have insisted on tests," she said. Instead, Anita accepted the doctor's diagnosis. On some level she really wanted to believe the doctor. After all, if he was right, she could make herself better by exercising, losing weight, and working less. So Anita went on a diet. "I lost ten or fifteen pounds over the next few weeks."

The weight loss that should have made her feel better didn't. "I just felt exhausted. It was an effort to get through the day. I would walk to lose weight, but it would wear me out very quickly. I felt hideous."

Since her days in the antiwar movement, Anita had always been active in politics. She had many friends in Milwaukee whom she'd often meet for dinner and parties. Lately, however, she didn't have the energy for much socializing. "If I wasn't too exhausted, I would go out and do things. But I found that I was doing less because I was tired all the time."

Still, Anita pushed through the fatigue and stayed as active as she could. Then came the afternoon of December 5, 2003.

It was holiday time, and Anita was getting ready for a festive party, bringing a few things to her car from her apartment. She was in the parking lot with her arms full of holiday gear when, suddenly, she didn't feel well.

"I became really short of breath. I couldn't breathe." She felt weak, nauseous, and exhausted, and she could barely move; she needed to sit down. Immediately, she knew this wasn't normal, nor was it anything she had felt before. Sure, she had been feeling tired the last few months, but this was at a whole different level, and it terrified her. "I was very frightened, because I had never felt that way before," she said.

Anita dropped her things at the car and staggered, huffing and puffing, gasping for air, back to the lobby of her apartment building, where she sat down. "I just couldn't make it back to my apartment. I was just sitting there looking forlorn."

Never one to cry wolf, Anita nevertheless took her cell phone from her pocket and dialed 911. This was serious.

In just a few minutes, four Milwaukee firefighters arrived. "Big strapping guys," is how Anita described them. The firefighters checked her pulse, which was 140, and her blood pressure, which was high. She was still having trouble getting air—she could barely breathe. She knew she needed to get to the hospital. It quickly became clear that the rescue crew did not want to transport this woman anywhere.

Anita said she'll never forget what happened next: the firefighters downplayed the seriousness of her condition. "First they tried to tell me it was anxiety. That made me more anxious. Then, they said I had the flu. One of them actually said to me, 'You should crawl into bed, and you'll feel better in the morning.'"

The flu? She couldn't breathe! She'd had the flu before, and this wasn't it; this was far more serious. And who were the firefighters to diagnose? They weren't doctors; they weren't even nurses. "I knew something else was wrong," she said.

Anita needed to go to a hospital, and she tried to convince the firefighters. But they pushed back. "They told me that it would cost three hundred dollars to go two blocks to the hospital. And I said, 'I have health insurance.'"

"Insurance won't cover this if it's the flu," they told her.

Anita wasn't worried about the money or the insurance. She needed help. "I don't care!" she screamed at them. She couldn't understand why they were being so difficult. After all, they were supposed to be there to help her.

Back and forth they went, but the firefighters wouldn't budge. "This went on and on," Anita said. Finally, she gave up. "Just go away," she told them.

Before they left, however, they required Anita to a sign a form saying she was refusing treatment. Reluctantly, she agreed.

Anita's experience with the firefighters still baffles her. "I have never understood this," she said. "I am a perfectly respectable-looking person."

The firefighters left Anita where they found her, in her apartment building's lobby. She still couldn't make it back upstairs. And she still knew she was seriously ill. So she stumbled to her car and drove herself the two blocks to Columbia St. Mary's Hospital in Milwaukee.

When she got there, she saw that the emergency parking lot was full. By now, she was having second thoughts. Maybe the firefighters were right; maybe her condition wasn't as serious as she thought. Anita decided to park in a distant lot. "Instead of driving up the circular drive and saying, 'Help me,' I parked a block away and started walking."

It was a slow, grueling walk. "I'd take a couple of steps and catch my breath, and then another couple of steps and catch my breath again." She looked haggard and was coughing. Finally, Anita spotted two nurses smoking outside the emergency room. She later thought how ironic: smokers coming to the aid of a heart-attack victim.

When they saw her, the nurses sprang into action. "I must have looked like Holy Hell," Anita said. "They ran to me with a wheelchair and whisked me in and screamed for a doctor. I didn't even stop for registration."

"They put me on oxygen right away and immediately did a chest X-ray," Anita explained. The X-ray revealed that Anita had double pneumonia. But the doctors weren't convinced that pneumonia was all that was troubling Anita. So they attached some leads to her and took an electrocardiogram

It was a few minutes before Anita got the results. She didn't think she had anything to worry about. She had pneumonia, which was bad enough. Then a doctor came in.

The cardiologist, Dr. Cornell Cohen, said, "You're having a heart attack."

Anita repeated the words to herself.

A heart attack? That didn't make sense to her. No, she was short of breath. This was in her lungs. He could be mistaken. "No, they said I have pneumonia," Anita told the doctor.

But the doctor was not mistaken. He knew what was happening. "The two are not mutually exclusive," he told her.

Pneumonia is, of course, a serious medical condition. In fact, it's the third leading cause of hospitalization in the United States, killing forty thousand to seventy thousand Americans a year. For those hospitalized with the condition, the mortality rate is 10 to 25 percent.

But what many people don't know is that pneumonia is often associated with heart disease. In a study published in the journal *Clinical Infectious Diseases*, researchers found that nearly 20 percent of patients who were hospitalized with pneumonia were also experiencing a major heart problem, such as arrhythmia, congestive heart failure, or a heart attack. And a study in *The American Journal of Cardiology* found that 28 percent of patients hospitalized for myocardial infarctions, commonly known as heart attacks, had recently experienced respiratory problems. Doctors think that respiratory infections like pneumonia can quickly inflame coronary plaques and even cause them to rupture, which can result in a heart attack. And a recent study suggests that pneumonia vaccination can significantly reduce the risk of death from a heart attack.

It's likely that Anita's heart problems were at the very least made worse by the pneumonia. "Pneumonia can trigger a blockage," she explained. "It can be the last little straw."

She was sick—so sick that Dr. Cohen wouldn't go home, even though he was missing a seder, a ritual dinner held during the Jewish holiday of Passover. "He was sure that his wife would forgive him when he told her how sick I was," Anita said.

The doctors at St. Mary's quickly performed an angiogram on Anita, and they found the worst possible scenario: her blockage was too severe for them to clear with angioplasty. She needed surgery, and she needed it immediately. But, the doctors told her, she was too sick for an operation. "They couldn't operate on me if I had double pneumonia because I would never come out of the anesthesia," Anita said. So they would have to wait a few days for the pneumonia to clear—hoping Anita would last that long.

There wasn't any heart disease in her family, at least not as far as she knew. And pneumonia? It was all so serious, so dire. And they needed to operate to clear her arteries. And it needed to be done now. But they couldn't, because she was too sick.

Anita was wheeled to a room in intensive care where, alone, she stewed over her predicament. She didn't call anyone, not even her parents or friends. She just couldn't bring herself to pick up the phone. "I needed time to wrap my head around it before I could talk to anyone," she said. "I just couldn't deal with my elderly parents."

Her hospital bed seemed so far away from them and the neighborhoods where she and her siblings had grown up in the late 1960s.

*   *   *

Anita Fox, a self-described "little red-headed girl," was born in Chicago. Her mother was a teacher and her father a Teamster for Borden Milk. There were three children, two girls and a boy, and shortly after Anita was born, the family moved to a farmhouse on the outskirts of Milwaukee. It was the middle of nowhere, but Anita liked the place. It was wide open, and there was a lot to do outside. "It was fun," she said. "We ran around in the fields." When she was older, the family moved to a home on a quiet street in downtown Milwaukee. "We had to walk a few blocks to catch the bus. It was pretty peaceful."

The peace ended for Anita with the Vietnam War. Like so many others who came of age in the late 1960s and early '70s, Anita was heavily involved in the antiwar movement. "I was a bit of a rebel. I was involved in the protest marches."

Although she was accepted to the University of Wisconsin and started taking classes, she wasn't there long. "I dropped out so that I could hitchhike across the country," Anita said. "I was madly in love, and he and I hitchhiked from Washington, D.C., to San Francisco." It was 1971, and Anita was twenty.

One driver took the couple across most of the country, from Washington to Colorado. There they bathed in the Colorado River before continuing on. "We had to hold on to each other so that we wouldn't get swept away," she said.

When Anita was thirty, she went back to school at Wisconsin and graduated with a degree in journalism. She worked a few jobs before settling into a position as a manager of e-mail marketing at the American Society for Quality, a not-for-profit organization based in Milwaukee.

Anita never married and doesn't have children, though it's not because she didn't want them. She hasn't yet found "the right guy," she said, and many of her long-term boyfriends turned out to be duds. "There were problems with infidelity," she said of the men she dated. She chides herself, however, for always falling for the wrong people. "You could put me in a room with one hundred men, ninety-nine of whom are the salt of the earth, and I would choose the asshole. Like a moth to a flame, I am drawn to bad, bad boys."

Besides not finding the right man, when she was twenty-four Anita lost an ovary, which left her unable to have the children she had always wanted. She grew close to her best friend's children, Velvet and Miles. Anita was in the hospital when Velvet, the first child, was born. "The nurse in the recovery room called me in, and the nurse asked me if I wanted to carry her over to be weighed and measured," Anita said. "So she handed me this little, squirmy baby." That's all it took. "I was in love," she said.

Then Miles was born, and Anita fell in love with him, too. "I always thought of Velvet and Miles as the children that I didn't have," she said. "They knew that they could come to me if they needed anything, if they needed help or to talk to somebody."

When Miles started having problems after his father died, he went to Anita for advice. Like any teenager, Miles would get frustrated with his mom, and he shared those feelings with Anita, too. "He trusted me," she said. It was a relationship less like a parent and more like an aunt. "He was the son I never had."

Two days after his eighteenth birthday, in 2002, Miles was killed in an automobile accident. It felt like Anita's own son had died, and she hurt deep down and all over. "I was unaware until then that grief is physically painful. It really is. I felt like somebody had ripped my heart out. That's what I imagine having your heart ripped out feels like. It was the worst."

After she heard the news, Anita couldn't think straight. "I was in shock. I once walked away from my car and left it running for two hours in a parking garage while I tried to arrange things to leave town for a few days. It was a terrible thing. I wasn't thinking straight."

Anita sought comfort in her friend, Miles' mother. "Her first words to me when I walked in after Miles' death were, 'I knew he was your boy, too.'"

Miles' death, and the times following the grave loss, took a toll on Anita's health. She had been overweight for some time, but she started eating more now. "It wasn't necessarily stuff that was bad, she said. "But I ate a lot, and that was bad. There was no portion control. I could eat a four-piece chicken dinner." Ice cream was one of Anita's weaknesses, and she'd eat nearly a whole container in one sitting.

"They started coming out with those Ben & Jerry's pint containers. That was evil," she joked. She could eat the whole thing.

*   *   *

Her first night in the hospital, Anita tried to come to grips with all that had just happened. When she came to, there was no family there: no mother, father, siblings, significant other. Eventually there would be the priest who'd come to deliver the last rites.

"Picture being alone in an emergency room after what I had been through. First they say you have pneumonia. Then they tell you you're having a heart attack, and they take you to a room where they stick a wire into your heart. Then they tell you that your arteries are too clogged for angioplasty or stents, and that you need open-heart surgery—but you are too sick to have open-heart surgery."

Anita was in a tenuous emotional state. She even began questioning her self-worth. The emotions went all the way back to the doctor who had told her months earlier that she was sick because she was old, overweight, and overworked. "My doctor yelled at me because I was fat," she said. Then there were the firefighters who wouldn't take her to the hospital. "They didn't think I deserved to live. It didn't make me feel like anybody cared."

She felt so old, so unattractive, so sick, and so helpless. "That's the kind of crazy thing that goes through your head when somebody won't help you," she said.

That first night, Anita was pumped full of drugs. "One of the things they do when you are having a heart attack is give you morphine," she said. "They don't want you to be in pain or to struggle against the pain, which could cause more damage." She was also given massive doses of antibiotics and clot-busting drugs. With all that in her system, Anita was a bit stoned. "I was flying high. . . . . [I]t was very surreal."

Anita got through the first night, and by the next day she was ready to call her parents. But how does a child tell her parents that she has pneumonia and heart disease and needs life-saving emergency surgery? "It's really hard," she said.

Anita decided to break the news to them in stages. First, she told them she was in the hospital. Then, she disclosed that she had pneumonia. Next, she snuck in the heart attack. Then she worked her way into the news about the delayed open-heart surgery.

Her parents, who both had health issues of their own, were soon at her bedside. They visited with Anita, making their own up-close diagnosis, as parents need to do, and then stepped outside the room to speak with the doctor. Only later did Anita learn what they had been told.

"The doctor told them that he didn't know if I would make it through surgery. He told them that I had a massive heart attack, and that with the pneumonia I was very weak, and he didn't know if I would make it." Her parents never let on what they knew. They were only positive. "It had to be devastating for them. My poor parents."

Anita was in intensive care four days. "I was unable to get out of bed or do anything," she said. Columbia St. Mary's Hospital has a chaplain service to provide religious guidance and support to patients and families in situations like Anita's. During her four days in intensive care, a number of clergy members visited Anita's bedside. Though she was heavily sedated, Anita remembers the priest best because she was raised Catholic, although she had stopped going to mass and openly practicing her faith years earlier.

She recalls that he was a sweet man in his 50s. "The priest came in and said he understood that I was really ill, and that he'd like to anoint me. But I didn't quite understand what he was talking about." Then the priest mentioned the sacrament of the sick. "Oh, my, that's the politically correct name for the last rites," she thought. Anita was terrified that she was going to die. "It was very hard. It's still hard for me to talk about it, although I am well past it."

Still, the priest was comforting. "When you are scared out of your wits, it's very comforting to have a priest absolve you of all your sins, even if you are a 'fallen away' Catholic," Anita said.

Besides the visit of the priest, another, more-powerful experience happened during those hazy days in intensive care. Anita has trouble explaining it, but it was a spiritual experience unlike anything else. She remembers lying in bed, being very cold, and being terrified that she was going to die. Suddenly comforting warmth enveloped her. "I had a feeling of peace come over me. And it was very warm and it felt safe, like being hugged by your mother. . . . It was all those things that make you feel safe." At the same time, Anita felt like she was outside her body. "It was like I was watching myself. I don't know if I was dreaming. I don't know if it was real or not."

Real or not, the experience had a real effect on Anita. She had renewed optimism, peace with herself, and felt comforted. For the first time since being admitted to the hospital, she was starting to accept her sickness. Also, and most important, she was no longer afraid to die. "It took that away. I don't feel like I am ready [to die], but I am not afraid. I don't think I will be afraid."

On December 9, 2003, Anita underwent beating-heart triple-bypass surgery. The beating-heart technique is relatively new. During traditional bypass surgery, doctors administer a solution that stops the patient's heart. A heart-lung machine then takes over during surgery, keeping the patient alive by oxygenating the blood and pumping it throughout the body. Because the heart is stopped, the surgeon can more-easily perform the delicate work of grafting new blood vessels. When the surgeon is done, the patient's heart is restarted.

Though traditional bypass surgery usually is successful, it can have complications. For instance, restarting the heart can damage the heart muscle, and it can cause arrhythmia or even a heart attack, especially with high-risk patients such as the elderly and those with extreme heart conditions.

Recently, however, a procedure was developed whereby surgeons don't need to stop the heart. It's done with a tool called a tissue stabilizer that immobilizes one part of the heart while the rest of the heart continues beating. In the beating-heart procedure, doctors don't need to stop and restart the heart, nor do they need to use a heart-lung machine.

Beating-heart surgery has been shown to have a better survival rate than traditional bypass surgery. That's because there is less chance for damage to the heart muscle, and fewer other complications. Patients also generally have reduced recovery times after beating-heart surgery, and they return home from the hospital sooner. Also, there is less chance they will suffer from "pump head," a side effect in which patients develop memory problems and other cognitive impairments.

Anita's surgery was a success, but like so many other people, she was afraid she would get sick again. "Right after a heart attack you are terrified that anything you do is going to cause another one," she said. "At the first sign of any twinge, I'd be like, 'What's this?'" Her doctor prescribed cardiac rehabilitation, which helped build Anita's confidence in her repaired heart. "It was the most wonderful thing, because I learned to overcome my fear," she said. "They put you on exercise machines, and they have you on monitors, and they taught me some wonderful relaxation techniques."

There were bouts of depression, but they didn't last long. Soon Anita's confidence was on the rise; she felt better physically and mentally, and she felt better about herself.

Six weeks after surgery, Anita had a follow-up appointment with her surgeon, Dr. Curtis Quinn, the same doctor who had warned her parents that Anita might not survive the surgery. A lot of doctors can be impersonal and unapproachable. Some, like the primary-care doctor who had dismissed Anita's symptoms months earlier, are downright insensitive. Not Dr. Quinn.

"I'll never forget when I went to see him six weeks after surgery," Anita said. When Dr. Quinn saw her, he couldn't believe this was the same women. He looked her up and down, and then glanced at his chart. Finally he said, "You look pretty wonderful." The words filled Anita will joy. "I feel pretty wonderful," she replied.

Anita's cardiologist, Dr. Cohen, was equally supportive. He was the kind of doctor who cared about his patients as if they were friends or family. It wasn't just medicine to him; he was interested in other aspects of his patients' lives. "He'd sit down and just talk to me for forty-five minutes before he ever bothered to check on my heart," Anita said. "He made me feel like somebody thought I would get better."

Just months before, Anita had thought no one cared whether she was alive or dead. Then she was surrounded by people who had confidence in her, were supportive, and wanted to help her get better. Anita felt like a new woman. "I could not believe the difference in the way I felt six weeks post-op. It was like my life changed."

Anita no longer sees the primary-care doctor who told her she was fat, old, and overworked. She thinks that the firefighters who wouldn't take her to the hospital dismissed her because she was a woman. They weren't educated about female heart disease, and that needed to be changed. Anita filed a complaint with the Milwaukee Fire and Police Commission. "Somebody had to know so that it didn't happen to another woman," she said.

Anita said the department was terrified she would sue. "The fire chief called and apologized for the shoddy care I received. And he did inform me that the four guys that came to get me were put through additional training so that they would recognize the danger."

Anita had considered suing the department but decided not to. She was happier than ever now. The entire experience helped Anita realize what is important in life. Now she takes more time to enjoy the little things, like spending more time with family and friends. Work is still important, but it's not the most important part of her life. "I work less than I did before. My co-workers and employer are wonderful, but they'll go on if I die. There's no point in killing myself for a job."

Anita also finds herself enjoying things she wouldn't have before— including exercise. "I never thought I would find myself happier if I exercise than if I don't," she said. "But I miss that little rush of endorphins [if I don't work out]. There's a good feeling that comes from exercising." In addition to doing Pilates and resistance weight training, Anita walks a lot, particularly in a hilly area near her home. "It's very challenging," she said.

Besides changing her exercise habits, Anita has changed her diet. "I eat strictly organic fruits and vegetables. And I reduced the amount of animal protein. I still eat meat, but not very often." Her portions are smaller, too. "Now I will have one piece of chicken, not four. And I have a scoop of ice cream, instead of an entire carton."

All that exercising and healthy eating was the key to Anita's weight loss. She dropped more than 75 pounds from the 270 she weighed. It's a remarkable achievement, but she isn't done. "I've still got a ways to go," she said.

With her renewed energy, Anita now travels more that she was able to before. "I've been throughout the West and the West Coast in the last few years." She's been to Yellowstone National Park, the Grand Teton Mountains, the Badlands of South Dakota, New Mexico, northern Wisconsin and Canada. She's also been to San Francisco to visit her friend's daughter, Velvet, who lives there. "I was walking up and down the hills like nothing," she said.

Anita has also been able to do some of the other things she loves, like being involved in politics. She was a volunteer for Hillary Clinton's presidential steering committee in Wisconsin.

It's an ironic consequence of a heart attack: Anita is happier and healthier now than she was before it struck. "I am a good survivor. I have a very full life. I am very lucky." And despite her near-death experience, Anita doesn't see her heart disease as a burden. "It was a good experience for me. I am content. I have a good life and friends. And a really neat second chance at life."

If you haven't been there, you'll likely have trouble understanding that—how having a heart attack can be a good thing. "People look at me strangely when I tell them that my heart attack was one of the best things that ever happened to me," Anita said. But what they don't understand is that Anita now knows what's important in life.

She wants to educate women about the symptoms of heart disease and encourage them to be assertive with their health-care providers. "The more women know about heart disease, the more insistent they will be," Anita said. Her reward is making a difference in other people's lives. "If I can make a difference for one person, it makes me feel pretty good," she said. "And I know I've made a difference with a number of people."

Anita still has pain in her heart, but it has nothing to do with disease: it's due to Miles's death. "You never recover," she said, "but the sharp edges get rounded off so that the grief isn't quite so fierce. And you still think with regret, but you also laugh about happy memories."

Perhaps the biggest blessing of Anita's experience with heart disease was a lesson she shared with her father before he died. He had been sick for a while, having been diagnosed with colon cancer fifteen years earlier and then undergoing chemotherapy, which damaged his heart. He lived fourteen years after that, but his condition worsened in November 2007.

On the last day of January 2008, Anita visited him in the hospital. He was in bad shape. "I sat in the room with him, and sat really close to the bed, and laid my head close to his, and talked to him for three or four hours," Anita said. Her father, deathly ill, talked back. At first they discussed practical things. "Don't let your mother spend a bunch of money on a dumb funeral," he said. "And get that car window fixed."

Finally he let out his emotions.

"He told me he was sorry that he wasn't going to make it," Anita said. "Daddy, you have nothing to be sorry for. You fought hard and lived a long life and have been a good father," Anita reassured him.

"Are you scared?" she asked him.

"A little."

"You don't need to be."

"Why?" he asked.

"Because people you love will be waiting for you, and you'll be safe and warm and healthy again."

"How do you know that?"

Anita thought back to her time in intensive care when she, too, was close to death, and that warm, peaceful feeling that overcame her and drove away all the cold and all the fear.

"Because," she said, "I was there."

Chapter 6:   Evan Kushner

The doors swung open and the emergency room team at Boston's Beth Israel Deaconess Medical Center sprang into action. Paramedics were handing off a patient suffering from an acute myocardial infarction, or MI—commonly known as a heart attack. This would have been a routine emergency—if that were possible—except that the patient wasn't the typical older male, in his late fifties or sixties.

The stiff but conscious figure on the stretcher was young, very young. Only thirty-three years old, and he appeared fit, lean, and muscular. It was Evan Kushner, a prominent Boston attorney, and he was just as perplexed as the Beth Israel medical team as to how and why he was in the ER and needing their help. Speeding-car accidents and drug overdoses are what usually drive young adult males to the emergency rooms in this country.

Evan was conscious, but not all there. He was pale, able to answer questions, and too afraid to ask what was going on.

The Beth Israel ER team was curious. They wanted some answers, and they needed them quickly. Their interrogation bordered on relentless. "Have you ever done drugs? What about cocaine"?

The young attorney didn't appreciate the cross-examination. He wasn't a drug user. "That just wasn't me," Evan said. "Even if I had tried cocaine only once in college, as a freshman, I would have told them."

There was no reason for him to lie. When you're flat on your back in the ER, denial is no help to people trying to save your life. That's the time to confess all your demons—especially those that could kill you.

Evan had no family history that could have put him at high risk for cardiovascular disease or a heart attack. There were no apparent external factors, unless you counted the incredible stress, much of it self-imposed, that came with his efforts to reach the top of the legal profession. Out in that world, a mere two hours earlier, the handsome, 6-foot-2, dark-haired bachelor had been the center of attention at his law firm's holiday party.

Evan is the founder of Kushner & Marano, a budding, mid-size practice that he started from scratch, just barely out of law school at age twenty-six. The holiday party was to be a chance to unwind. Kushner & Marano had invited its young office staff to Jillian's bar and Lucky Strike Lanes, behind historic Fenway Park. It's one of those places where Boston's young, well-heeled professionals gather to bowl, dance, drink, see and be seen.

The party numbered about fifteen, half of them lawyers, half support staff.

Some peeled off to go bowling. Others disappeared in the entertainment megaplex, looking for drinks or a Boston Celtics game on one of the plasma-screen TVs.

As he scanned the bar, Evan could have been recalling that while he was a self-made man, there had been some breaks that eluded the other young lawyers and MBAs gathered here. For starters, he didn't leave Suffolk Law School in downtown Boston having to repay student loans that usually climbed well into six figures. His father, a successful businessman, had paid his full tuition. So the money he made would be his free and clear once he finished law school.

Evan had been a good student, working for the law review and finishing near the top of his class. His plan was to become independently wealthy by age forty, and that meant working hard and long hours in the meantime. Divorce cases, real estate, civil suits—Evan handled everything. He wanted and needed the work.

"There was no trust fund waiting for me," he explained.

Evan always went to bed with a radio or TV turned on "because if not—my mind races." He kept a pad and pen in the bed so he could make notes of casework that needed to be done. This went on through the night. Even if the power was out, Evan said, "I'd fill up half a pad. My mind just continued to race."

And he was up by five most mornings.

"Get up, get my coffee, depending on what was going on maybe go to the gym or go straight to work. The pre-9 o'clock hour was so valuable because the phone didn't ring. It was about getting through stuff."

He often put in a full day's work on Saturdays. "I'd go for my coffee, I'd read the paper, and I'd work. On Sunday I may work two hours or I may work twelve. Sometimes you get in the flow and you are productive and you enjoy it, and I can just run the table."

The more he produced, the more he was rewarded. From the start he was billing clients $125 to $150 an hour. "As you get busy, the fee goes higher and higher. Now, I bill out at three-and-a-quarter."

This young attorney was working killer hours, but he wasn't trying to kill himself. A frequent visitor to the weight room, he watched his diet and his waistline. He wasn't a smoker or much of a drinker. He didn't need any compulsions outside of work. Besides, cigarettes and booze didn't fit the image he was crafting of one in control at all times.

It was always important to be seen as the first rather than the last to leave a party, and the holiday gathering was no different. On the night of his heart attack, Evan had an associate give him a ride home, early. His condo in fashionable South Boston near Back Bay was but a ten-minute drive from the bowling alley.

Evan went to bed, and then the unthinkable began to happen.

"I can't tell whether I was starting to fall asleep or what, but I felt a cramp in the middle of my chest. It was one of those where—sometimes you just kind of stretch your rib cage and it goes away. It felt like a muscle cramp."

The former power forward for Newton South High School's basketball team was accustomed to temporary minor aches and pains. A banger under the boards, the teenage Evan Kushner often caused as much pain as he took while helping lead Newton to the Massachusetts state championship game, which it lost to Wakefield High.

Then there was college at the University of Massachusetts at Amherst. His game wasn't big enough to attract a scholarship offer, but Evan took his brashness as a banger to the campus courts, where he went toe to toe with students who had honed their hoop skills on Boston's rough inner-city playgrounds and public high school gyms.

That's where Evan first discovered that he may have been sheltered in Newton, a predominantly upscale Jewish suburb of Boston. Evan recalled one incident during a pickup game while he was at UMass: he was stunned by a sudden fist to his face in the midst of a heated argument with a bigger, tougher, and angrier student from Boston's Broughton area.

As with that fist, Evan said, he could not have imagined the cause of the sudden cramp inside his chest. But this was different. This punch lingered and twisted around in a place where it should not have been, where it couldn't be massaged or iced.

Evan decided to call his best friend, Jay Werner, who happened to be a doctor, a radiologist. He got a recording to leave Jay a message. Evan made a second call, to his mother. "I felt very much in control at this time, but I had the elephant on my chest. It hurt. At this point, it is not dawning on me that I might be having a heart attack, just that something's wrong."

It took a mother's plea to convince him that he had to seek help, and that the time for gathering further opinion and deliberating was over. "Go to the hospital" she cried. "Call 911. We'll meet you there."

Evan had more questions. "OK, shall I drive?"

"No, call a cab."

He'd gotten a verdict, but the young attorney wanted to poll the jurors. He was looking for consensus. Was there anyone else he should call? Could this be something other than an emergency?

Evan was running out of time. He didn't know it, but the longer he delayed getting to a hospital, the greater the odds he could die on the way or in the ER. This was no time for his deductive legal reasoning to take over. Beth Israel, one of the best hospitals in Boston, was just a mile down the street, but if he didn't get there in time, it might as well be in the Middle East.

Evan called Jay Werner again. This time he answered.

"My chest is killing me. I woke up and it's killing me," Evan said. Jay would later say that his good friend sounded very scared.

"Hang up the phone and call 911," Jay screamed into the phone. "This is your heart. You don't fuck around with it." Jay rarely used such language, but he knew his friend had to get moving or he was going to die.

Evan obediently made the call, finally.

"Hello, I've got chest pain," he said. A 911 operator had picked up the phone after the first ring. The dispatcher began an interrogation.

"Have you been drinking or doing drugs."

"No," Evan said. He could hear the dispatcher directing an ambulance to his home. "We've got a thirty-three-year-old male complaining of chest pains."

"You can hear the communication go back, and it didn't seem like it was happening to you," Evan said later.

"Sir, someone will be there shortly."

Evan put on sweatpants and a sweatshirt, collected his wallet and keys. A faint siren grew louder, signaling that help was on the way and paramedics would soon be at his side. He unlocked the front door and left it open, and then positioned himself at the end of the bed as the rescue workers entered.

"I don't know if the first thing they gave me was morphine or the nitroglycerine," Evan said. Whatever it was, they asked him if it was relieving the pressure. Evan wasn't sure. They checked his blood pressure a few times.

Then something happened, something small but something that let Evan know—if there was still any doubt—that he must be in trouble.

"At one point, the way my apartment was configured, I needed to go a matter of six feet—they couldn't get the gurney in. And I was like, 'Guys, I can do it.'"

"'No, don't do anything, they insisted.' Things like that start to be of concern. I still thought that I was under control. I still could have a conversation. I wasn't in so much pain that I couldn't think straight."

But there was that elephant still sitting on his chest.

As Evan was being wheeled down his steps into the ambulance, his parents pulled up, their faces full of fright. They had already been to Beth Israel and could find no record of their son having been admitted. Fearing the worst, they rushed to his condo.

"As I was getting wheeled into the ambulance, in the driveway to my apartment building, I saw my parents pull up and get out of the car. And

I've got a mask on; I've got stuff taped to me. And—I am sure you can relate to this as a parent—through the mask I can't say, 'I'm OK.' And that's what they see until we get to the hospital."

The trip to the hospital was quick, and Evan was now in the ER. "They are doing different things. They are trying to give me different things for the pressure to go away. I felt like I was in there for two hours. It wouldn't surprise me if it turned out it was forty minutes. Eventually, the pressure subsided."

The hospital staff at one point suspected Evan might be suffering from pericarditis, an inflammation of the thin, membrane-like sac that contains the heart. The cause of pericarditis is unknown, but it can be acute or chronic.

It would be hours later, with all the data now returned, that the hospital staff concluded that Evan had suffered a heart attack.

"So, I'm in intensive care. That morning there was something in the newspaper, and I am more comfortable now. I think I am OK. I called my law partner to discuss the newspaper article, but I didn't mention that I was in the hospital. I thought I was going home in the afternoon."

"So they are taking more blood tests and doing the EKG, and they've done an echocardiogram, and now the enzyme is starting to show up in my blood. What they found was that on the interior part of the heart, I had an artery that was completely blocked. In fact, I had an MI." A heart attack.

Doctors decided to go into the artery with a wire and balloon to unclog the blockage, then insert a stent to keep the artery from closing again. The stent is a tiny, wire-mesh tube that is mounted on the balloon and carried through the artery to the damaged area. It's a common and effective procedure; more than a million are performed in the United States every year. Patients with multiple blockages sometimes have more than one stent inserted during a single procedure.

Evan had been lucky. Anyone who survives a heart attack—mild or massive, even at age thirty-three—has to be considered lucky. But this young man was hardly in the clear. There would be other scares, more emergency trips to the hospital, and three more stents inserted into his arteries before his forty-second birthday.

Evan would never have his life back the way it had been, which is not to say he would not have a lot of good living ahead of him.

The stent itself is not overly intrusive. The required slit in the groin where the wire and balloon are inserted is perhaps the biggest nuisance. Once the hemorrhaging from that slit has stopped and the cut is stitched or stapled shut, the patient is discharged and told not to do anything for a few days.

Evan was home a mere two days and nearly going out of his mind from boredom. "I went to the office and said to my receptionist, 'I'm not actually here.' It was the end of the year, and I had stuff to do. You know, I felt as though I was accomplishing something."

Many heart-attack survivors are encouraged to participate in cardiac-recovery programs. Evan lasted about a half-hour in his hospital's wellness program.

"I was half the age of everybody in there. Everybody else was overweight and trying to quit smoking. They all fell into the category of people we expect to have heart attacks." What he meant is, they were old.

"It was people like that. I have nothing in common with these people. To sit me on a bike . . . I couldn't do it—it was depressing."

So Evan checked out. "I made one appearance, and I was off to my own devices. I knew it as soon as I walked in. But at that time, you want to do everything that is available to you, like what will make me better."

Alone and without a support group, which is what the other patients in cardiac rehab could have been, Evan experienced the emotional roller coaster that typically comes with surviving a heart attack.

"My initial reaction after everything settled down was, 'Why me?'" He was angry, but he also thought, "Thank God I didn't die. First and foremost, I was really, genuinely appreciative."

In the back of his mind, however, was the resentment from knowing that thirty-three-year-old males are not supposed to have heart attacks. Evan didn't want to be seen as being sick by his friends.

Some figured Evan's illness was work related because, "I was going a million miles an hour. My cardiologist said that just isn't it. I had other friends who said, 'Forget it, I'm not going to keep working out and exercising, because you work out much more than I do. You're in much better shape than all of us. If it happened to you, there are clearly no boundaries.'"

"I stopped lifting weights for strength and tone," Evan said. "I had to slow it down there, and I had to change my cardio workout. Eventually basketball was no longer a great exercise for me because of the stopping and the starting, the sprinting. So I had to do other things that kept my heart rate up at a good level."

Evan bought a heart monitor and often kept it on during the day under his clothes. He started counting each stair he climbed during the day, and weighed each decision on when to take the elevator. It took Evan nearly two years to figure out how to approach his world of work differently. But what's two years when you're planning to spend at least a few more decades, and hopefully more, on the planet? Someone suggested he work at an 80 percent pace, but he couldn't do that. If his motor had six gears, Evan couldn't downshift to fourth or even fifth. He enjoyed speeding too much.

So he decided to take on less work. "I could turn away work and still work at 100 percent. But I can't work 80 percent on all that work. Because my mindset as a young lawyer trying to grow his practice is, 'I want all the deals.'" His life goals hadn't changed much after the heart attack: he wanted to work, and he still wanted to be financially independent by the time he was forty.

Evan talked to a therapist, but he wasn't willing to surrender control to anyone. He politely refused direction from the therapist. "I was like, 'Why don't we wait and see what happens. It's still my personality. Let me solve things on my own.'"

"I had anxiety issues, probably about three or four months out—couldn't sleep and breathe comfortably—so I went and talked to someone, and it didn't particularly help, but I was open-minded to anything and everything."

The shield of invincibility that many young men feel never totally returned for Evan. The heart attack had robbed him of that.

"You start to gain some confidence in things, but as I got two, almost three years out, I'm thinking, 'You know what, it was an aberration.' Nobody said to me, 'Listen, you did this, you did that, or any of these things [to cause your attack]. We can't tell you why it happened.' So you begin to think you can kind of write it off. Be smart, eat well, exercise, do what you are supposed to do, and you're good."

Then came Evan's second brush with death, a reminder that if his body sent him another warning sign, he had better listen, or there might not be a third chance.

It was the end of summer 2002, and Evan was playing in a softball tournament in Virginia. He had become unusually tired. His friend Jay was there, on the same team. They had played four or five games over a couple of days in eighty-degree heat and lots of humidity.

"And I said, 'Man, am I tired.'

"Jay said, 'Make sure you hydrate.'

"I said, 'It's not that. I shouldn't be this tired.' But I had no pain or anything. And a couple weeks go by, and I'm shooting a basketball just by myself at the gym, and I am going after a rebound, kind of jogging over, and I felt a burn in my chest. I stopped playing, and as I walk around, I noticed as I walked briskly the burn picks up, and as I slow down it goes away."

This was different from Evan's first heart attack.

"The original heart attack was an elephant on my chest. This was just a burning. At the hospital, they would ask if I ever had indigestion, things like that. And I look back, and before the heart attack I never had any of those things. I never had reflux, anything. So, any pain I had there I assumed might have been muscular—overdoing it—but nothing ever stood out. So this burning was new."

Evan now knew his body far better than most people know theirs. When is a pain just a pain, and when is it heart related? Evan phoned his cardiologist. It had been almost three years since his heart attack.

"We set up for another stress test, and we had a couple of doctors there, and they have the EKG set up. I had been doing probably thirteen minutes or so on the stress test, which the reports say for a male of my age was pretty good. But I had to stop after seventeen minutes."

Doctors decided they would insert a catheter with a tiny camera attached to see if another blockage was causing Evan's pain. Their hunch was right.

"They found an artery that was almost 90 percent blocked, and there was a small artery that they would keep an eye on," Evan said. You've got lots of different arteries, and some are so small they close themselves up and regenerate."

Another stent was inserted, so now Evan had two in two separate arteries. "I now have limitations, and before I had no limitations. That's why I say the invincibility, it never returned. I couldn't run through walls anymore."

It was a position no one in his family, not his father or his grandfathers, had faced. The cardiovascular disease that was causing his arteries to harden and clog was his alone. It couldn't be blamed on his family's DNA.

The young lawyer had to take three more weeks off. Then it was back to the real world. Evan returned to work a different man. He was more reflective. There was a greater sense of the here and now. His quality of life needed re-examination.

"When I look back at those long work years, my social life suffered. I lived with a girl for a couple years a few years back, but that's been it. There has been lots of fun, and interesting dating stories, and girlfriends here and there. The relationships would last three months or six months; but not much longer.

About seven months after the second stent was put in, Evan had a follow-up stress test. "I probably run fifteen minutes, and I'm like, 'You know what, great! Everything is good.' But they saw something in the flow of the [obtuse marginal] artery they didn't like. So they decided they wanted to stent that one. This was in July of '03, and this was the first of the drug-coated stents. This would be stent number three."

This third stent may have been the most difficult for Evan. "I was not myself. I was out of sorts for days . . . meaning like a week. I wasn't remembering stuff. I couldn't stay focused on anything. I needed help to keep me focused. Now it just seems like it's just a bad respite. A few months go on, and you get past that, and I get back to my routine of doing stuff and living life."

But Evan's routine, his center, was different. It had to be because of his fragile health. Now there are a handful of times in the course of a month that something goes on and he will stop to check his pulse, or immediately go through a mental checklist. "You might feel your heart race, which happens to everyone. I become aware of my surroundings. What's going on? How long does the pain last? If the pain lasts a minute, I need to make a phone call."

He carries nitroglycerine pills with him everywhere to help open an artery should it close. Every day he must take the statin Lipicor, an aspirin, and a beta blocker. The plan is to keep the cholesterol low, the blood flowing through the arteries. It would be a good plan for most people with cardiac disease, but it doesn't seem to be working for Evan Kushner. There is something unique about the hardening of his arteries that the best doctors have not yet figured out. Still, they believe that keeping him on the medication regimen is a good precaution. And Evan has agreed to make himself available for new experimental treatments.

His fourth stent followed a Friday night incident. Evan was walking home about five blocks after having dinner with a friend and had to slow down about five times because the familiar burn would hurt so much. "I knew something was wrong . . . but I was like, 'OK. I caught it, I saw it.' I was looking over my shoulder. After three or four years, I thought I was kind of due for something."

The warning pain had become both a blessing and a curse: a sign to get to the hospital to be checked out, and a reminder than he had a medical condition that would forever haunt him—if he let it.

The Kushners have always been big sports fans, and Boston's professional teams were on a roll around the beginning of the new century. When the Red Sox won the World Series in 2004, Evan was there. When the New England Patriots and quarterback Tom Brady were winning three Super Bowls, the Kushners were in the stands.

The family had been season ticket holders to Celtics games, going back to the championship days when magnificent players like Bill Russell, John Havlicek, Sam Jones, and Larry Bird would take to the parquet floor of the Boston Garden, and coach Red Auerbach, in the beginning, would light up a cigar right on the bench when the team had the game well in hand. More recently the Celtics had fallen on hard times, until 2008, when they again reached the conference and NBA Finals.

"I missed one of those Celtics games because of the fourth stent," Evan said. "I was in such a depression. My head was spinning. I wasn't ready to hear the, 'Listen, you detected everything, you are in tune with it, you're good, you're gonna be fine.' I know that's people being supportive, but I couldn't hear it."

"[Then they] had that game seven against Cleveland; it was a three-thirty game. I didn't have any interest in going, but my dad is seventy-three now, and it's a real opportunity to watch it with him.

"We go to the game and I watch, although there is not much of an expression on my face. The energy of the crowd was so unavoidable. And it's not like I stood up and cheered, but it was so infectious inside me. The buzz you get when you walk out of a game and your team has won. Certainly a game like that took me out of the doldrums and at least brought me up to 'miserable.'"

There had been attractive women in the row behind Evan. As he and his dad were leaving, one of them asked him if he was from Cleveland. She figured as much because Evan appeared to be dejected, as though his team had just lost the game.

Evan explained that he had been a diehard Celtic fan all his life. It's just that on that day he was not capable of displaying any emotion but despair.

"I couldn't manifest anything; I wasn't trying to pretend to be happier than I was. But I know it brought me from dark and gloomy to something above that."

Living with cardiovascular disease is a process. Some days are better than others. Evan expects that a fifth stent will be needed at some point, but the key is learning how to pack a lot of living in between those episodes.

When he travels abroad, he researches what coronary care is available, especially in developing countries. "East Africa is not as good as South Africa as far as access to medical. I'll go to East Africa now because doctors were just inside [my arteries], and they saw the other stents and everything there looked good, all my other vessels looked good."

"They just got their best look, so I think this is the best time to do it. Give me two or three years, and I will be looking over my shoulder again."

Evan said he now feels "a greater sense of urgency to do things. There are so many times that people want to have meetings, and then they want to schedule a meeting for something else, when nothing has been done. If I schedule a meeting we have a to-do list, and I don't want to meet again until we actually do those things. Life is too short. My time is too valuable."

"Sometimes you just gotta buy the ticket, because if you don't buy the ticket, there's always gonna be something that comes up."

"I have friends in New York. In the past, if I could only see them for a day, it wasn't worth it. But now it is worth it for a day, and I've done that. Coming down to D.C. Whatever it might be, it's making the time. And I am fortunate that I have a professional life that allows me the freedom."

"I have people at the law office to hold down the fort. I have that type of freedom. I don't want to be the guy that had the opportunity to do things all this time but never did it. People have said to me, 'You have a bucket list.' I hadn't thought about it like that, but kind of."

"I had an opportunity to go to the Playboy Mansion in March. A friend of mine knew somebody that sponsors the Playboy golf event."

So Evan visited the Playboy Mansion.

"I'm going to Costa Rica. I am traveling for about a week and a half, and then volunteering in San Jose. I am going to work at a soup kitchen and an orphanage."

"That's about being the person that you want to be. I want to be somebody that gives back. I want to be somebody that my nephews look up to, and I have the time to do that and to be those things."

"Part of picking East Africa is that I'm trying to get involved with something . . . maybe on an ongoing basis in Kenya. I'd like my trip to be about me, and then be about something that is not about me. That's the person I want to be."

"I think I can do a few things that might be able to help a bit more. So I'd love to find an organization that can make good use of that. I'm a bright, capable person. You can show me stuff and not have to worry that it won't get done. Not everybody is that easy."

Chapter 7:   The Reverend James Love

If you want to know

where I'm going,

where I'm going soon.

If anybody asks you

where I'm going,

where I'm going soon.

I'm goin' up yonder.

I'm goin' up yonder.

I'm goin' up yonder to be with my Lord

Walter Hawkins, Goin' Up Yonder, 1976

The blue-and-gold-draped choir members at Evangel Temple swayed and rolled like waves on a deep sea. Their voices were two hundred strong, backed by a full orchestra with horns and guitars. On this Sunday morning, the music was so loud and joyful, it might have awoken angels in heaven.

It was September 8th, 1996, and one thousand five hundred parishioners packed the church, many of them standing and waving to the music. The congregation was frenzied because one of their own—a boy who had been raised in the church and was now a respected pastor in Greensboro, North Carolina—was returning home to deliver the 11 o'clock sermon.

To the congregation, the Reverend Doctor James Love was no longer another kid from the tough streets of Southeast, Washington, D.C. Now he was a respected man of the church, a man who escaped a life in the projects and made a name for himself in the church and in the communities where he worked. Everyone was excited to see him return home.

When he was growing up, James was always hanging around Evangel Temple. His mother sang in the choir, and she'd bring him with her, by bus, across town to the church, which back then was on Rhode Island Avenue in the city's northeast quadrant. While she sang, James played with the other children.

It had been many years, but James's mother still sang in the Evangel choir, and she was there the day James returned.

"How that boy had grown!" she exclaimed.

At 6-foot-1 and 270 pounds, James was an imposing figure. And at age thirty-nine, by the standards of the church elders, he was still a young man. But despite his relative youth, the bearded, brown-skinned preacher with a soft yet firm voice had a reputation for "bringing down the house."

"That Sunday is indelibly imprinted on my mind," James said later. "I was excited to be preaching in the church where I grew up and knew so many people."

It was a wonderful occasion for James to come home, and he imagines how excited his mother and the others must have been to see him return. "Think about this. Here is your son going away. He's grown up. He's got a family. You invite your son back, and you are proud of him," James said.

And it wasn't just his mother who was excited. This church in this community was like an extended family. "Everybody in the church is your mom. They are your uncles," James said.

As the 11 a.m. sermon neared, James's adrenaline was pumping. He put everything into his sermons. Whenever he preached, he spent the day before sequestered in the church's study, reviewing Scripture, practicing out loud and praying.

James didn't just preach with his words. He communicated with hand gestures, the pitch of his voice, and his body movements, many of them spontaneous, sometimes uncontrollable. He was often so animated and intense during his sermons that afterward he'd be drenched in sweat. He always kept fresh shirts nearby.

James didn't want that homecoming at Evangel Temple to be any different. He planned to inspire his church family, many of them elderly, many facing economic hardship and family problems. He stayed up all night preparing.

His sermon would be based on the Gospel of Luke, Chapter 22, Verse 34: "I tell you, Peter, the cock will not crow today until you have denied three times that you know me." James titled his sermon "But I Prayed for You." The message would be that Jesus is there for us even when we, like Peter, have lost faith.

Though the sermon reflected his Christian beliefs, neither he nor Evangel Temple is tied to a specific denomination. James, who describes himself merely as "a preacher of the Gospel," said many denominational churches are losing members because of their socioeconomic and religious structures.

"People feel comfortable here because here we do not have a particular denominational DNA," he said. "You know you are in a Roman Catholic church, you know you are in a Methodist church, because of the rituals and the rites that they have. Some people are comfortable with that tradition. Other people say that there's got to be more than this." He said nondenominational churches like Evangel Temple provide much of the experience of a denominational church—the messages, praise, and experience with God—without the rituals and liturgy.

Nonaffiliated churches like Evangel Temple have grown over the years by drawing Christians who had been labeled Baptists, Methodists, and even Catholics. You can see the popularity of such churches on TV every Sunday.

Evangel Temple outgrew its inner-city location years ago and moved to several acres in Bowie, Maryland. Every Sunday the church is packed—even the overflow room. There's so much demand that the church provides DVDs of its services to those who can't make it on Sunday or don't arrive early enough to get a spot.

James wanted his homecoming sermon to be something to remember. He wanted to leave the congregation with renewed vigor for the Lord and Evangel Temple. His sermon started just as planned that Sunday. The congregation was alive and excited. It was just as he had hoped.

"They were in the aisles. As the young people say, I'm pumped. I'm coming home. And I'm gonna preach and I'm gonna pray until the glory cloud comes down and people are moved. And not just moved from an emotional standpoint, but that they really get the message and respond to the message. I must have really prayed and prepared myself. I was ready for this."

On the way to the temple from their hotel room that morning, his wife, Deborah, had noticed that James didn't look normal. His color was pale, his stride a bit off. "I didn't want to push him too much," Deborah said. "But I did get him some juice."

Not long after, James started his sermon, preaching to the packed church. It went well, until halfway through.

"I was standing in the pulpit, nearing the end of my sermon, when all of a sudden I started sweating profusely. I became nauseated and dizzy and exhausted. But I kept preaching."

He felt like he was carrying a set of dumbbells while standing in quicksand. His body became rigid. He was no longer able to raise his arms. His mouth continued to move slowly, but he could no longer hear his own words.

"I knew I couldn't go on," he said. "Pain was starting in my chest like an elephant was sitting on my chest. I signaled for the pastor, as an invitation, to take my place and finish my address."

James staggered off the pulpit and flopped into his seat.

"I stumbled. There were some steps going up the platform to the podium. I went down and hit the last step and remember stumbling just a little bit, and one of the people kind of steadied me."

To the congregation it looked like Reverend Love had just worn himself out. Southern preachers were famous for collapsing, even falling unconscious, after bringing the church to a fit with a stirring sermon. Sometimes it was real. Other times it was part of the show. But this was far more serious; his words and his balance should have been dead giveaways.

"I had never cut a sermon short before," he said later.

Deborah knew there was a problem immediately. After sixteen years of marriage, she knew when James wasn't being himself. "His language, his movements, and his hands—everything was out of character. His cadence was off. His pitch was higher than normal. He appeared peaked."

Deborah quickly and quietly moved from her seat to within whispering distance of the church's leader, Bishop John Mears, an elderly, thin man and heart-attack survivor from years past. "Something's not right," she whispered to him. Deborah knew she had to do something, so she moved from Bishop Mears to a couple of deacons and insisted they help James off the stage and into the church's office.

"I sat down," James said, "and they were fanning me and giving me water. I continued to be listless, lethargic."

They all thought James needed something in his system. He was given cookies. No one called an ambulance, and no one suggested he might be having a heart attack.

"I am thirty-nine years old! Heart attacks are for people in their sixties and seventies. So they thought I was just maybe a little tired," James said later.

Instead of going out to dinner that night as planned, the clergymen and their wives decided to go to the house of Bishop Mears, who lived in a nearby gated community, so James could lie down. But he still didn't feel well. It was nearly forty minutes after his sermon, and he still felt a pressure in his chest and was sweating profusely.

Deborah still blames herself for not recognizing James's symptoms earlier, for not insisting they go to a hospital. "I knew the signs," she said. "I asked him if there was pain in his arm, an elephant on his chest. He kept saying, 'No, no.'"

For a while it seemed James was improving. The he suddenly grabbed his chest in pain.

"Oh, my God. He's having a heart attack," Bishop Mears said. Coming from the bishop, it must have sounded like a revelation. Someone contacted Dr. Hector Collison, a prominent Washington cardiologist who was Mears's neighbor. Collison said to get James to the hospital immediately, and he would meet the patient there. Within minutes an ambulance arrived and rushed James to nearby Prince George's Community Hospital. Deborah followed in their car.

The emergency medical technicians started treatment in the ambulance. "I got a little relief from the nitroglycerine I was given in the ambulance on the way to Prince George's," James said, "but the real relief happened when I was taken from the ER to the cardiac-intervention lab."

At the hospital, a doctor broke the news to James. "I was asking him what was going on with me, and he said, 'Sir, you are having a heart attack.'"

His reaction to what the doctor said made no sense, he later admitted.

"Will this take long?" he asked. "I have a flight to catch."

"Sir, you're going to be here for a little while," the doctor responded.

It's been said that people responsible for helping others—clergy, doctors, and teachers, for instance—can have a difficult time admitting their own frailties or accepting medical treatment. That was certainly true for James.

"I was messed up emotionally. When I was in the hospital, in the emergency room, I said, 'Lord, what's going on here? What is wrong with me?' I really didn't believe that I was having a heart attack. I associated heart attacks with obese people, or people who were older."

The experience caused James's faith to waver, despite his years working in the church, even despite his message of faith to the congregation a short time earlier.

Dr. Collison arrived at the hospital to perform an angioplasty. He explained to James exactly how they would proceed. As Collison spoke, it dawned on James that he was in serious trouble. He was having a heart attack. "Do what you have to do," I told him.

Dr. Collison threaded a wire into James's arteries and discovered two clots in his right ventricular artery. He cleared the clots by inflating a balloon attached to the wire, pushing the deposits against the walls of the artery. Dr. Collison had performed the procedure, called angioplasty, in hospitals throughout the area hundreds of times.

"They didn't put a stent in," James said. "I was awake. [Dr. Collison] was talking to me."

The pain was gone almost immediately.

"I remember I was breathing a lot easier, like the weight just fell off of me. It was just wonderful."

James was moved to a hospital room with a single bed. Though he was feeling better, the minister struggled privately with his emotions. "How can I have a heart attack? This is not supposed to happen to me," he thought. "Why didn't anybody pick up on the signs?"

Though doctors disagree on the exact role stress plays in heart attacks and cardiovascular disease, most think it's a contributing factor, if not an outright cause. James is sure stress played a role in his sickness. An admitted Type A personality, he was always on the run and always had more to do than the hours in each day allowed.

James's path into the stressful ministries had begun years before, on the rough-and-tumble streets of inner-city Washington where he grew up. It was a place, he said, where a kid's innocence was lost fast. When James was in just fifth grade, a girl in his school was raped, and his school was locked down while police searched the grounds.

"I remember the police everywhere," he said.

His teacher asked James if he knew what rape meant.

"She explained it to me, and I was quite horrified," he said. "So, I grew up in a kind of a rough environment. But we didn't know it was rough. We didn't know that was the projects. It was all we knew."

There was more than just crime. This was the 1960s, a tumultuous period for America, particularly in the country's inner cities. James remembers when Martin Luther King, Jr. was assassinated. "My community is in an uproar," he said. "And the National Guard was called out and stood guard literally on every street."

It was a time of chaos and rioting.

"They literally burnt that whole section of community out," James said. "These were mostly business owners who were African-American. This was a black community, and we burned our own [businesses]. I never understood that."

James's family moved out of the District of Columbia to nearby Prince George's County, Maryland, in 1968, at the beginning of a massive black flight from the city. Similar exoduses took place in many other major urban areas around the country.

"We moved into an apartment complex just over the D.C. line that was all white," James said. "We were one of the first black families to move there." But as black families moved into Maryland, white families moved out. "That community changed from white to black literally in the blink of an eye," he said. "The white families ran from us. They moved into Landover and Bowie, Maryland."

It was a firsthand experience with the troubled state of race relations in the country. "That raised a whole sociological issue with me with respect to race relations," James said. He wanted to learn more. He wanted to know why white people didn't want to live near blacks. After all, he had white friends at his suburban school. *What was going on?* he wondered. It was a question that stayed with him.

Immediately after college and seminary studies, James became a novice preacher at Evangel Temple. He was assigned to work on community issues. "We were dealing with the issues that the urban community has to deal with, and I was just fascinated by that," he said.

James was trying to find answers to big questions such as how churches in urban communities can help solve problems like homelessness, teen pregnancy, unemployment, crime, and school dropouts. That led into his doctoral study.

"My thesis was that the urban church is the citadel of the community, and that the urban church cannot afford to just do religious things. We cannot have what I call a 'hand-out ministry.' We gotta have 'hand-up ministry.'"

James thinks the answer lies in education. So while he was at Evangel Temple, he started GED programs, homework clubs, after-school care programs and mentoring programs.

An experience with a homeless man convinced James that the church needed to do even more. The man asked James for money. "I looked at him and I said, 'I'm gonna do one better. Let's go into McDonald's and eat. Let me buy you something to eat.' I wanted to hear from this guy. So I bought him something to eat, and I said, 'Talk to me. What's going on? How can the church be more responsive to helping you in particular?'"

James was moved by what the man told him. Churches really don't care about people like me, the man told him. They don't have programs. Church people just pass us by. They look at us as not even being human, as being just things.

That experience convinced James to expand his efforts. "Jesus says, 'I was hungry and you fed me.' Now, I don't have the money to take care of all poverty. But we do have a moral obligation to say, 'What can we do to alleviate some of the suffering and some of the misery?'"

James concluded that the church's soup kitchens and clothing banks weren't enough.

"A lot of the programs, all they do is provide a handout," he said. "The fact of the matter is, if you don't teach me to fish, I'm always dependent upon you for fish. And so if you teach me to fish, I can fish for myself. I won't be dependent upon you." James also wanted to help latchkey kids, youngsters left home alone by their parents. It gave him the idea to work with parents to provide after-school programs for children. Basketball clubs, for instance. Safe, structured places where children could go to get off the dangerous streets.

"Your kids can come here for a couple hours until the parents come home," James explained. "[We can] work with them, with their homework. The carrot [is that] they get to play basketball. The church has an obligation to do that. I just believe that it is our responsibility as a church to reach into the community and provide empowering programs."

In the early 1990s, James moved to Greensboro, North Carolina, from Washington to work as an associate pastor at Christ Covenant Church. He also ran a private Christian school of two hundred students from preschool through grade eight. "Education is kind of my thing," James said. "So we went down there and had a wonderful time."

Running the school was a big job, involving working with parents and fundraising. In addition, James was a husband and a father of three: twin daughters and a son. "My kids were young, so I was also involved in the things they were involved in," he said.

James dived into his adopted Greensboro community. There were meetings—lots of meetings—to attend. Folks looked to James for advice and saw him as someone who could get things done. "Reverend, can I talk to you about something?"—that was the beginning of many conversations that lasted hours. At the same time, James was working on his dissertation for a doctorate.

James admits that while he was dividing his time and attention in a hundred directions, he was ignoring his health, probably taking it for granted. "I was a little heavier than I am now. I was carrying a little bit more weight than I needed to."

He did get some exercise. He always loved basketball, and like most boys who grow up in the city considered himself pretty good. Every Thursday he played with a church group, but that wasn't enough cardiovascular exercise to keep him healthy, fit, or stress-free.

"So I got all these things going on, so there's stress, stress," James said. "And I didn't take vacations. I thought that was a waste of time. Why would you take a week off? Maybe I would take Friday and come back maybe Tuesday. For me, that was a vacation. That was all you needed."

James said he was working hard because he wanted (and perhaps felt he needed) to make a difference in other people's lives. But it was too much for him. "I was taking on so many different things. I wasn't really relaxing" or sleeping, he said.

The drive to improve the lives of those in his community at his own expense is a quality not unique to James. In their drive to help others, many ministers often ignore their own health.

"The tendency of clergy, for the best of reasons, is to be self-effacing, to take care of others before taking care of yourself," said Rev. H. Gray Southern, who in 1993 oversaw nearly one hundred Methodist churches in the Durham, North Carolina, area. "You're the 'suffering servant.' You're the 'wounded healer.' It's hard to set boundaries."

The health of clergy has become a growing concern. In 2007, the Duke Divinity School in Durham was awarded $12 million by the Duke Endowment for a Clergy Health Initiative, a program aimed at assessing and improving the health of "every United Methodist pastor in North Carolina," according to a July 2007 school news release. The program, which will involve health coaches working with clergy members on such matters as diet, exercise, smoking, and behavioral changes, is a response to studies on clergy health in recent years.

"The initiative will employ practical steps toward improving the health of clergy, who have been shown in various studies to have one of the highest death rates from heart disease of any occupation," the news release said.

According to a Jan. 7, 2009, *New York Times* article, the program has conducted focus groups with ninety ministers and staff members, and surveyed one thousand eight hundred pastors on health issues. The results of the study will be released in academic papers over the next two years, the Times said.

James Love would have been at risk for a heart attack had he not become a minister. If recent studies are correct, James, like most African–Americans, was born at risk. Those studies show that heart disease strikes more African-Americans at a younger age than previously thought. A March 19, 2009, article in *Time* magazine referenced a study published in *The New England Journal of Medicine* showing that one in one hundred black adults develops heart failure in his or her thirties and forties, "a rate 20 times higher than that of similarly aged white men and women." The study also found that blacks often don't receive treatment for high blood pressure, which contributes to heart disease.

"The end result is that African-Americans are more likely to develop further risk factors for heart disease, none of which are being treated aggressively enough to protect this population from early illness," *Time* said.

Like others with heart disease, James did have a warning.

In Greensboro in 1995, he had felt his jaw lock and then felt paralysis across his shoulders and couldn't move his arms. It lasted about ten to fifteen minutes. James went to the emergency center at Moses Cone Hospital and was given an electrocardiogram, or EKG, which turned out to be normal. The doctors said he was dehydrated, and released him.

Some doctors won't let a patient they suspect may be having a heart attack leave a hospital even if the EKG is normal. Many doctors believe EKGs are far from a perfect means of detecting a heart attack. In December 2008, for example, another thirty-nine-year-old man, Edward Givens, was given an EKG by paramedics who went to his home in Northeast, D.C., not far from the original site of Evangel Temple. The fire department rescue team concluded he was suffering from acid reflux and told him to take an antacid for indigestion. Six hours later, Givens died of what the medical examiner concluded was a heart attack. Relatives later revealed there was a history of cardiovascular disease in his family: his mother had survived a heart attack in 1994.

James didn't see any doctors about his heart health. He remembers that he occasionally had physical examinations, but they never revealed much. One doctor told him that he had borderline high blood pressure and needed to monitor it. "I didn't really watch it," James admitted.

Though James wasn't too concerned about his health, his wife was. In fact, she sensed he was working too hard, and she turned to the Lord for help. "I said, 'Lord, it's time for you to do something,'" Deborah explained. "'Don't kill him. Just shake him up a little bit, because it's time for him to slow down.'" A month later, they flew to Washington for the service at the new, bigger Evangel Temple in Bowie.

Like many heart-attack survivors, James insisted that his attack turned out to be a blessing. It forced him to look at how stress impacted his life. He had to slow down and re-evaluate his purpose for being here. But perhaps most important, it allowed him to let other people into his life who could help him.

After his heart attack James returned to Greensboro. He took Dr. Collison's advice and enrolled in a comprehensive cardiac-rehabilitation program at Moses Cone Hospital. "It was physical rehab. It was counseling. And you met with a dietician," James said. "You work on stress and things like that."

Unlike many other cardiac-rehab centers, the one at Moses Cone had lots of young people, James said. "There was a young lady there who was in her late twenties. The thing that struck me about her was that she was so young. And the others that were there were probably in their mid-forties. There was nobody old. When I say old, I am talking sixty, seventy."

There was a routine at the cardiac center. "The first half hour, they took our blood pressure, pulse, and all that. Then they told us to get on the treadmill and do a couple things like that," James said. "And after about a week of that, you went to see your counselor, who talked to you about how you were feeling." The next phase focused on diet. "The dietician—he helped me! The fried stuff has cholesterol, and the cholesterol blocks arteries. [They] talk about carbs, all that kind of stuff."

Giving up his favorite foods was a challenge for James. "I love ice cream. I am known as Mr. Ice Cream," he said. "You wanna bribe me? Put some Breyers butter pecan [in front of me], and I'll do whatever you want me to do. I had to recognize that this stuff was killing me. Slowly, deliciously, it was killing me."

The food at all the church dinners was to blame, too. African-American churches are renowned for great home-cooked meals, and the health of an overweight minister is never questioned by the church community. Who would dare suggest he's a heart attack waiting to happen? It would be heresy to question aloud the health benefits of home-cooked meals.

After his heart attack, however, James became a convert, promoting heart-healthy home cooking. His wife actually led the way, but James followed. He knew that his life and the lives of his flock were at stake. It was important, James thought, that the African-American church family change what they cooked and ate, and how they looked at food.

James's church in Greensboro was predominantly white. "There is a difference in the way a traditional white church [prepares its meals]—regardless of its denomination—and a traditional black church." He said that in his experience, "white churches usually have balanced meals. There will often be fried food, but there will also be vegetables and fruit.

"Now, in a black church, after an event . . . there's gonna be a lot of fried stuff there. You're gonna see fried chicken. You're gonna see ham. You're gonna see fried fish. You gonna see all kinds of things, fruit, vegetables to some extent; grits, macaroni and cheese, a roll with butter." The drinks served always included iced tea with sugar, he said.

Deserts were no healthier. "Apple cobbler, peach cobbler, maybe a pound cake. If Mother so-and-so baked a pound cake, of course we gotta have a pound cake."

James said that the unhealthy food served at African-American churches is part of the culture, part of the religious experience. "I think it's part of our cultural DNA," he said. "There were certain foods that we had access to, mostly pork and things like that. And I think our grandparents taught our parents, and our parents continued that same tradition."

"Unlike traditional white churches, we knew how to celebrate even in the midst of pain and struggle," James said. "There was always that kind of celebration, even in the midst of sadness. I think that we carry that over, particularly at deaths, at births, [and] at points of celebration."

"There was always food present."

James is convinced that if enough preachers lead, their congregations will follow them to a different kind of buffet. "We're killing our preachers," he said. "I ate whatever I wanted to eat. Like most ministers, too much fried stuff. Fried chicken [and fried] fish. Pizza."

In 1997, James left Greensboro to become a pastor at Faith Tabernacle United Holy Church, a Pentecostal congregation on Capitol Hill in Washington, D.C. "Fried food galore," he said of the new church. But James doesn't eat all that high-fat food anymore. His wife makes sure of it.

"I no longer allowed him to eat at church," Deborah said. "I prepared all his meals. Everything they did was fried or buttered at Faith Tabernacle. Fried chicken, fried fish, fried okra."

The meals Deborah made at home were heart-healthy. "I was preparing baked skinless chicken, and cooking his vegetables with broth instead of pork and grease," she said. And his new church community helped Deborah keep an eye on her husband. "Even if I wanted to have fried chicken," he said, "there would be a deacon or a mother in the church to say, 'Pastor, you don't need to have that.'"

The culture at the church started to change. "People started thinking differently," Deborah said. "We started bringing people in to talk about eating heart-healthy. We convinced them that healthy people could do more for the Lord."

Soon there were healthy options at Faith Tabernacle meals. "We changed the culture a little bit from the heavy emphasis on macaroni and cheese, and fried food, to more fruit, vegetables, chicken," James said. "Baked chicken and fish were alongside the fried stuff."

Many larger African-American churches are changing, Deborah said. They cater a lot of their meals, and there is a good balance with baked foods and salads. It's the smaller congregations—those that don't have the budgets and must rely on volunteers—that continue to cook the old, dangerous ways.

Sometimes James spoke about heart disease to some of the older men in the church. He would encourage them in all aspects of health. "Get your prostate checked," he would tell them. "You need to check your cholesterol. Take a walk."

And James didn't pretend he was without faults. "I would say to them that I am not perfect in this. I have stumbled."

James also told them that physical health is related to spiritual health, which he said too many people disconnect. "If you are obese or overweight, if you're smoking, or drinking, or addicted to certain things, it's going to hinder your spiritual ability."

James remembers his discussion with one man who was overweight and didn't think there was anything he could do about it. "I would talk to him straight. Person to person. Privately," James said. "As a pastor, I can say certain things that other people can't say."

He brought that message to many of the folks in his church. "In a general kind of way, [I] encouraged people to be heart friendly, healthy. You don't have to be extreme. Park your car a little ways away from the mall and just walk. Do things like that, things that you don't think about. It makes a major difference."

James doesn't preach good health from the pulpit with the passion that accompanies his sermons on the Gospel. That would be going too far, he said, causing church members to look around and identify who's fat and who's fit. James and Deborah would rather lead by example than edict.

"We haven't, as ministers, always seen ourselves as living examples [of health] because we've been overweight," James said. "We have just eaten whatever we want. But I think more and more of the younger ministers—and I am fifty-two—guys in my age group, are much more health conscious now than [were] my mentors."

James said he thinks of the heart attack as "my second birth. I think God was saying to me, 'There is still work I have for you to do.'"

He also thinks it was a warning, a lesson. And he's changed nearly everything about his behavior as a result. "If I get tired, I'll rest a little bit. I don't sweat a lot of stuff now. I really don't." And unlike before, James now takes days off. "Every Monday I'm off," he said. "Unless you [are] dying, don't call me on Monday. Period!"

And he takes a month-long vacation every August to Williamsburg, Virginia. "Before I had my heart attack, I never had time for vacations. In fact, I thought they were a waste of time. Now my wife, who is a teacher, and I make sure we get away to coincide with her breaks from school. It's important for us both."

Exercise has become a part of his life, too. "Now I exercise religiously. Three to four days a week, I walk for forty-five minutes on my treadmill, and I do some modified weight lifting," he said. "I'm proud to say my lifestyle changes have rubbed off on my children. They are all healthy, and my son, who is now twenty-six, is training for his first marathon."

James's mindset changed, too. Before, he said, his competitiveness made him his own worst enemy. Take basketball, for instance. "I often said that if I was just a few more inches, I'd probably be in the NBA. I was serious. I'd play basketball [for] four or five hours in the snow or in the rain.

Everything was a competition for James, even everyday tasks like mowing the lawn. "We may be friends, but the bottom line is, I'm gonna mow it faster than you, better than you," he explained.

He used to be competitive in his preaching, too, but not anymore. James said he realizes that's not the right mentality. "I've had to learn that grace over the years, and I think I'm there," he said. "I still have a little bit of that competitive thing. But I think that [my] heart attack helped me to put things in perspective. It helped me to see that my life was more than a compilation of things to do."

James's schedule isn't like it was before, either. Before his heart attack, he kept a list of things to do, broken down by month, week, and day, and he would track his progress. At the end of the week, James would calculate what percentage of his tasks was completed. "A 70 percent week was good," he said.

He no longer sweats the small stuff. When James feels stress, he stops counseling people. He puts the cell phone in a drawer. He takes time off. "People either deal with it or they don't." he said. "It's not arrogance. It's realizing there is a God, and it's not James Love."

James still preaches, at his own church, Love the Word, in Prince George's County. He also teaches three classes at a local community college. But James now knows his boundaries. If he is late grading his students' papers, for instance, he asks the dean for an extension. He no longer beats himself up over it.

"'No' has become one of my favorite words," he said. "If I'm asked to do something that doesn't fit my mission, I respectfully decline. If there is someone else who could do something just as well and often better than me, I've learned to ask for help and to delegate. I take time to appreciate each day, and I always put my family first."

James has a different perspective on his higher mission, too: he now realizes he doesn't have all the answers to America's racial and urban

Chapter 8:   Mary Maguire

In April 1993, Mary Maguire had a heart attack. She was forty-six, and as incredible as it might sound, Mary had no clue what was happening to her. Heart attacks are what killed the men in her family, not the women.

It was a Thursday, and Mary's day had begun like the one before it and the one before that. It was always the same routine. She didn't like sudden changes or surprises.

"I never had a driver's license, so I was waiting for my husband to pick me up after class in his truck." Mary was studying to become an operating room technician.

The couple lived in Wheeling, West Virginia, a town of about thirty thousand in the northern part of the state. The residents of Wheeling seem to have divided allegiances among three states because of their proximity to Ohio and Pennsylvania. Bethlehem, Pennsylvania, once famous for its steel plants, is not far away. Pittsburgh is the closest big city, and most of Wheeling cheers for that city's Super Bowl champion football team, the Steelers.

As for Wheeling, it's home to the Kruger Street Toy and Train Museum, which boasts an impressive collection of tens of thousands of operating trains and toys. The layout changes frequently. The local Chamber of Commerce promises a nearby gift shop and coffeehouse will help round out your visit.

Try as she might, Mary couldn't hide the anguish in her face as her husband, Jim, pulled up to the curb. "I must have looked bad, because he asked if I needed to go to the ER. I said I didn't know." Not waiting for an answer, Jim pointed the truck toward the emergency room. Mary never wanted to be a problem.

"We had finished our clinicals, and then gone to lunch at Long John Silver's," she said. It was on the way back to class that the pain emerged out of nowhere, "stomachache, sweating, arm aching, really nauseated."

"All the signs were there," she later acknowledged. "Our class was on the third floor, and the elevator was down for repairs. We had to walk the three flights of stairs, and I remember stopping several times and telling those with us how bad I felt. They all just laughed it off."

Mary wasn't tall or lean. She was about 5-foot-3 and stocky. Her fatigue could have easily been written off by classmates as her simply being out of shape. With her classes, a husband, and a house to keep, who has time to work out?

"Once in class, we always had our lecture first, then a twenty-question quiz. I kept telling everyone how bad I felt, and asked if anyone else felt sick, too. I really thought I had food poisoning."

Mary said she was able to answer the first two questions on the quiz, but couldn't concentrate on the rest of the exam. "I was always one of the first to hand in the quiz papers, but I was one of the last ones still there, and wanted out of there bad, so I just circled anything without even trying to read or concentrate on anything."

As she and Jim now headed for the hospital, Mary worried that a trip to the emergency room would take hours out of Jim's evening routine, which probably included a beer and dinner in front of the TV. So she decided along the way that the pain, which came with a shortness of breath, was dissipating, and that she no longer needed acute care.

It was not a smart decision. Getting to an emergency room during a heart attack can often mean the difference between living and dying. Women and men are notorious for putting off the trip until it's too late.

"By the time we got close to the hospital, I was feeling fine," Mary said. Jim didn't insist that she be checked out, a second mistake. So they went home.

"I cooked dinner, cleaned up, washed clothes, and did my homework," Mary said. "Back then, I wouldn't go to bed with a dirty dish in the house, or clothes either for that matter."

She was accustomed to getting a mere two or two and a half hours of sleep every night. "There was always something I needed to do. My theory back then was, I'll rest after I die." It almost came to that.

That night after she went to bed, the pain returned as though it had been hiding, waiting for the right moment to pounce again. Mary didn't move. She was either too afraid or in total denial about what might be happening to her.

"It was back again, so I laid there and thought happy thoughts." Like the job she would get after completing her classes to become an OR technician. How to spend that first paycheck. "I wanted to buy a Christmas tree that touched my ceiling."

By Friday morning the pain had lessened, again proving that it could be cunning and baffling to a woman who didn't have the time to be sick. "I decided then I was really in control. That next morning, I went to clinical classes, and then missed my ride home, so I walked home, about three and a half or four miles. I was fine. But that night, again, when I finally got to bed, all the pain was back. But this time I couldn't control it at all. It would not go away at all."

Rather than lie down, or reach for the phone to call for help, Mary went to work in the house, watering the forty flower pots in her living room, some of them seven feet tall. She referred to the plants as her rain forest. "When I started to water them, I was really very short of breath, and it took a long time to get them all watered."

She had to know something serious was going on inside her. Self-medication became her first option. "I started taking aspirin. I took several; they didn't work, so I took more and more. Finally, I knew I had to do something. Jim was asleep, so I went to get him up."

Maybe he was in too deep a sleep and didn't hear her plea, or maybe he recalled the earlier trip to the emergency room the day before that she had aborted. "Go back to sleep, and we'll see how you feel in the morning," he told her.

She followed his instruction, but the pain lingered.

She thought about calling a neighbor for help but decided against waking someone else in the middle of the night. Mary just refused to be a bother, even if it meant her own life was at stake.

"So I just sat there and prayed," She said. Jim eventually woke up at 5 a.m. Saturday and drove her to the emergency room—but only after taking a hot shower before leaving the house.

The pain and the trip to the emergency room could not have come at a worse time, Mary thought. After raising her two children and spending most of her adult life as the supporting housewife, and sometimes working small outside jobs, she was about to become an operating room technician, a full-time, working contributor with skills. OR technicians made good money and were always in demand. Mary's self-esteem grew as she neared graduation.

"I had about two weeks to go before graduation, and then six weeks of internship, and I'd be a new person. I had a choice between two hospitals for my internship and knew whichever one I chose, I'd be hired. For the first time, it was about my best interest."

*   *   *

All of her life, Mary Maguire had been told she wouldn't amount to much. For the longest time she believed it.

Mary was born and raised in Martins Ferry, Ohio, just across the Ohio River from Wheeling. They lived in her father's parents' house, Mary said. "My parents took care of them."

"My grandfather died when I was a few years old. I can remember going to Sunday school and church a few times with my dad and grandmother. But mostly I remember my grandmother as being in bed for what seemed like a long time. I can remember going to her room and climbing on her bed and her scratching my back and telling me stories."

It had been a quiet neighborhood, where everyone really looked out for each other. Her father was a plumber, as was his father, and he had his own business. Some of the neighbors worked for Wheeling Steel, others were coal miners. The miners came home from work filthy, and Mary was glad her dad wasn't a coal miner.

"Back then we walked or rode our bikes everywhere. We went outside in the morning and stayed outside till the street lights came on. We were never home, but always in a neighborhood group together."

Her first exposure to death came when her grandmother passed. "I was a junior in high school; my whole world was then turned upside down. She went to the hospital the day President Kennedy was shot. She had a blood clot in her leg; back then, they just put you in bed and turned a heat light on it. Anyway, her phone rang, and she got out of bed to answer it and bumped it and fell. She never came back around after that and died in December before Christmas."

"She was in really bad shape, but I was forbidden to go see her. But after school, I went to the hospital and snuck into her room. I was real quiet. She had tubes everywhere. I started to cry, and it was like she was talking to me, but at the same time it was totally impossible. All I could think of is how she loved to make us all homemade doughnuts every Saturday, and homemade noodles for chicken soup. Everything had to be done on Saturday, because Sunday was her day of rest and to read her Bible."

"I knew I'd somehow be OK, and she would always be watching over me" after she died, Mary said.

"A few weeks after my grandma passed away, my grandfather got on a Greyhound bus and went to New York, got married and brought the woman back here with him. Sad part was, she looked enough like my grandma to be her sister. But the woman drank beer and smoked, which my grandma condemned a woman doing. She even sat on the porch in her chair. I hated her. She hated me, too, and for my graduation gift wanted to give me a one-way ticket and bring one of her own granddaughters over here in my place. She died several years later of cancer. I was not sad."

"My grandfather continued chasing women and wanting to get married again. One day he said someone was coming from Cleveland to meet him, and they were getting married. He had taken all his money out of the bank, and when my uncle got home from work, he went in and found my grandfather beaten up and all his money gone. He died several months later, probably as a result of the beating."

Mary grew up with two sisters and a brother. She's the oldest, which might help explain her obsession with taking care of everybody else and not having time to get sick.

"My sister is thirteen months younger than I am, the other sister is ten years younger than I am, and my brother is five years younger than I am. My sister that's thirteen months younger than I am, my mother always dressed us like twins, and for years a lot of people thought we were twins."

What Mary never shared with anyone was the humiliation she suffered at the hands of her mother.

"Growing up, my mother always called me stupid and dumb and retarded. So naturally, I really thought of myself as such. Even when she'd leave us kids alone, she would leave my sister in charge. She had all the brains, she said. All during my school years, my mother told me if I was real lucky, I might be able to work in a five-and-ten store, because you didn't have to be real smart to work there. I really wanted to be a nurse, but it was just a little dream of mine that I never dared to tell anyone, for fear of being laughed at, or teased about it."

"At the end of my freshman year of high school, I went to the rest room before walking home. My mother always taught us to never, ever use a bathroom other than the one at our house, even at school. Anyway, I went in, and when I was ready to leave, there was a retarded girl in there, and I asked a friend what was wrong with her, and she told me. I then asked if I acted like that, too. She laughed at me, and I cried. Then she told me no, and asked why I asked. I just said never mind. When I went home, I went to the bathroom, locked the door and stood there, looked in the mirror and really looked at myself. I also made some faces, too. Then I decided right there, no matter how long in my life it took, I was going to be a someone, I was going to make a difference, and I was going to be OK. But above all, I wanted to prove her wrong and make her proud of me."

It would take Mary years to keep that promise to herself. Martins Ferry High School had a vocational education department, and her mother made her apply for the cosmetology class. "Needless to say, that was the last place I wanted to be. But I had no choice. I made it into the class, hated it, and spent both my junior and senior years there. After that I was forced to go onto Wheeling Beauty College to qualify for a West Virginia license. I then worked as a beautician."

While working at a local beautician's shop, Mary met her future husband. "Jim and I, we went out for the first time on Mother's Day and were engaged in November and married in February."

"Back then, I made $35 per week, and I had to give my mother $25 per week, for room and board. Also, on my days off I had to clean her house from top to bottom. When we told her we were getting married, she was really mad. At first she said I couldn't get married till after my sister got married. On top of all the money I was giving her, I also had to buy my dress, my sisters' and my mother's dresses."

Mary and Jim found an apartment in the Warwood section of Wheeling. "Then I again changed jobs and worked at a wig shop styling wigs," Mary said. "I stayed there until our daughter was born. We lived in a mobile home for four years before buying our house we still live in today. Both our kids were born while we lived there. Living in a mobile-home park was fine as long as we were both working. But when our daughter was born, I became a stay-at-home mom. Our son was born seventeen months later."

After their children graduated from high school, Jamie enrolled at West Virginia Northern Community College, and later West Liberty State College. Bill went to Ohio Northern University to study pharmacy.

He later phoned his mother and mentioned he could get more financial aid if Mary was also in school. Bill challenged her to do something about her persistent complaints of not having the time or opportunity to go to college. He was adamant, and Mary finally agreed to accept his challenge. In the end, it was a serious mishap involving Jim that pushed her to enroll in the medical program.

In 1972, Mary said, Jim hurt his hand at work on the midnight shift. "When they called me, I knew it was bad, because he let them take him to the hospital and not come home first. It was there we met Dr. McConnell, a plastic surgeon, and I became fascinated with surgery. This man was incredible. He did fantastic things. Anyway, Jim ended up losing two and a half fingers. He was in the hospital for six weeks, with all the plastic surgery.

From then on, I wanted to be in the OR. I found the surgical technology program and started taking classes."

*   *   *

Mary's heart attack in 1993 meant that her dream opportunity, the OR technician position, would have to be deferred.

"We get to the ER, as I walked in, all the pain and discomfort went away. I was ready to leave, but they insisted on me getting checked out. Fine, I was OK, so that wouldn't be a problem.

"Well, they took a blood test, which showed I did have a heart attack. I would have to stay. To make matters worse, they put me in coronary care. No phone. Boring! Just rest and stay calm.

"Here I am getting ready for graduation and an internship, and they want me to stay calm. I told them I'd stay till Monday a.m., and then I was checking out and going to class. They agreed."

Mary was angry. Now she decided to be a bother to lots of people. She wouldn't cooperate with her medical team. There would be no surrender on the part of this patient. She fought them. Her cardiologist tried to explain the gravity of her situation—clogged arteries and maybe even permanent heart damage—but Mary wasn't listening.

"I threw books at him. He learned to duck real well, and eventually started to send nurses in to get the books before he would come into the room."

"Back then, after you had a heart attack, they made you wait a few days before they would do a catheterization on you. When they eventually took a look inside my arteries with the dye and camera, it showed all my blockages."

For the first time, in her mind, there was now proof of what the doctors had been telling her. Mary was in real trouble. Her own medical studies told her she could die if she didn't control her feelings of disappointment, while allowing doctors to begin trying to save her life.

It was a hard lesson to learn, that life can sometimes be unfair. It would eventually take angioplasty and quadruple bypass surgery to save her. And all the while, that dream of becoming an operating room technician was evaporating.

"I knew I was in real trouble," Mary said. "Then I started to make pleas with God, like, 'If you get them to let me be OK till I finish school, then I'll get checked out.' Lots of things like that. Like I was *still* in control, knowing I really wasn't. It was pretty bad."

"I threw things, fired doctors. Everything and anything that wasn't what I wanted to hear, that was my way of dealing with it and yet still be in control. I knew better, but it sure made me feel better thinking I was the one in charge."

Her cardiologist took the weekend off, which had nothing to do with Mary, but she was convinced otherwise. Eventually it was decided she would be transported to Pittsburgh for surgery.

"When the cardiologist came in and told me what hospital I was going to and where, I just said, 'OK. Now, leave me to do what I have to do. I need to change and rearrange my calendar all around.' Our dog we had at the time was on allergy shots, and I needed to change her appointment."

"I needed my hair cut bad. I also didn't want to wait till I got home, for fear of getting a hair in an incision and getting an infection. I had phone calls to make to let people know where I'd be.

"They then sent this Catholic nun in to talk to me. She meant well, but I'm not Catholic, and she had no idea how to deal with a control freak, let alone what to say to me. She said to me, 'Now, you know when you come home you won't be able to do laundry, vacuum,' and she went on and on. Finally, I said, 'Please, I have things I need to get done here, and you are stopping me. Please leave, right now. I really don't care what I won't be able to do, I need to think of what I have to do right now!' She left and told the cardiologist I had no clue what was happening. Yes, I did know, but I also knew what all I needed to do right then.

"I wanted my hair cut before I left. I had no idea what was in store for me, and I know I'm miserable when it needs cutting. I called Karen, who always cuts my hair, explained the situation, she came and cut it in the hospital." An ambulance or emergency car was waiting to transport her to Pittsburgh immediately after her hair was cut.

If there had been time, Mary might have gotten her nails and toes done as well. Mary told me that no woman wants to enter a hospital not looking her best, regardless of her illness.

Heart disease ran in Mary Maguire's family. Her grandfather once had a stroke. Of the three uncles on her father's side, one had a heart attack and open-heart surgery; another had several heart attacks and two open-heart surgeries. Mary said her dad suffered a heart attack and was driven to Cincinnati for an angioplasty when the lifesaving procedure was still fairly new. He died of a massive heart attack in 1994, the year after Mary's attack.

Still, heart attacks among the Maguire women were considered nonexistent when Mary was struck.

"They had told me I really had a lot of blockages, especially for someone my age. They also said it was my choice to have the surgery or not, but if I did, it might buy me a year or two at the most, and they couldn't guarantee my quality of life either way."

What choice did she have? She chose the surgery.

"I was in surgery for over twelve hours. During that time my family never heard one word. Finally, one of the surgeons came out to talk to another family, and my husband asked what about me. He told him they had finished two different times and had to reopen me both times."

"After my heart surgery, right after I got in my regular room, I was really sad. I just looked at my legs and my chest incisions and wanted to cry, they looked so bad and were all back and blue, too." Mary's legs were bruised because doctors took arteries from her legs to use in the bypass surgery.

"Anyway, in the midst of all this, every time I turned on the TV set, the little Energizer Bunny came on, and they kept saying he keeps going and going and going. I hated that rabbit! Even threw things at him. Finally, after this was happening several times, I decided there was a lesson here, and I had to figure it out. Then it hit me: after open-heart surgery, you have to keep going and become like that bunny, and just keep going and going and going."

Mary spent the next day and a half in intensive care. Her children came to visit her. She said Jamie had a hard time with it, as they all did. This mother and wife had always been the one doing everything for all of them.

Jamie was pregnant at the time, Mary said. "Because she is a diabetic, she had to see specialists in Wheeling and Pittsburgh. She had an appointment in Pittsburgh that day and was to come to the hospital to see me after her appointment."

Bill was there, too. He was always the talkative one, but he just stood in the back of the room saying nothing. Jim just stood there crying.

"Jamie stood closest and kept telling me she was having a girl. She told me over and over again. I started counting. She must have been really scared, because later she only recalled telling me once."

"For the longest time after I came home, Jim could never say 'No' to me, no matter what I asked for. It really got old."

Weeks later, Mary had an appointment in Pittsburgh with the cardiologist who had performed her multiple-bypass surgery. "He asked me what I wanted to do, and I said, 'Go home and cut grass.' He asked what was stopping me, and I said, 'You.' The doctor told me to go for it.

"First thing, I got my driver's license, and got up one morning, washed clothes, cleaned up the house, cut grass, edged the lawn, washed my car, got cleaned up and went to the mall. I was bored."

As for why Mary had never had a driver's license:

"When I was about to turn sixteen, my mother told me not to even think about driving, because I was too stupid and would only cause wrecks. So needless to say, I never mentioned [getting a license]. When my sister turned sixteen, my dad was out there with her every day [teaching her to drive], and after she got her license they even bought her a car. To make me feel better, she told me it was our car to share."

"After I had my heart attack and while I was in the hospital recovering from my open-heart surgery, all I could think of was what I would do if this would ever happen to Jim? How would I get around, and how would I get him to appointments? That's when I decided I had to get my license. After I was home for several weeks, I walked down to the state police office and got a book to study for my permit. The following week I took the test and passed."

After her heart attack and recovery, Mary went back to repeat some OR technician classes. But she would never work in an operating room; it turned out to be far too much stress. "I did go back . . . and finish my degree. I lost a lot of my self-confidence that I had before. I really think that it was because everyone was really watching me, just waiting to see if I was really OK or not."

"It was one of the hardest things I ever did, going back. The real reason I went back is, someplace along the line, Jim had said that all the guys he worked with had bets that school was a phase I was going through, and I'd never finish."

"After my heart surgery, he told me that, and then said, 'You're not going to finish now, are you?' Well, I had to after that. I graduated in 1994, a year later.

"My dad had passed. I went back to school following his funeral. During my internship, the OR team had a rough night, and I decided then I couldn't be an OR tech. When I get tired, I made and make mistakes and can't think real fast. In the OR, you can't make mistakes. So I never worked there."

She did get a position in a hospital as a coordinator in the Mended Hearts program. "It was my job to meet with all families as their patient was having heart surgery. I kept them informed of progress and updates, and told them when it was safe to leave and eat, make phone calls, etc."

West Virginians like to eat, and that usually means deep-fried, high-calorie, well-seasoned, Southern-style cooking with all the trimmings. Before her heart attack, Mary's diet included lots of red meat, fried foods, potatoes and homemade gravy. There were sodas and lots of junk food, especially when she studied or watched TV. Like many people, Mary felt a sense of entitlement to such treats after a hard day's work, or at weekend gatherings among working-class friends.

"Before my heart surgery, I wasn't a breakfast person; if anything I'd have [soda] and a doughnut or breakfast roll, or something like that, if anything. For lunch, it was mostly fast foods, anything at all, really. For dinner, I was the kind of ho-hum person who knew what was for dinner by the day of the week: Monday was always baked steak, mashed potatoes, and corn. Tuesday was either a pork roast or pork and sauerkraut. Wednesdays was spaghetti night, Thursday was either pork chops or meat loaf, with scalloped potatoes, and baked beans. Saturdays was hamburgers and French fries. Sundays was leftover day.

"Snacks were always junk food of any kind, and lots of candy, too, anything to help stay awake and get everything done. That was the goal. Then on Monday, we'd start all over again. Ugh! Amazingly enough, I never considered that boring at all. Scary today."

During her recovery, Mary learned what her original cardiologist was trying to teach her—that major lifestyle changes had to be made. That while heart attacks are the leading cause of death for women as well as men in this country, many, if not most, of those deaths can also be prevented. Diet and exercise are keys, she told me.

"Before my heart attack, there was no time for exercise, or even the thought of it at all. For several years after my heart surgery, I belonged to a fitness center, until it got way too expensive, then I bought a total-body-workout bike." Mary said she used to use the bicycle every day, but has been slowed recently because of a torn meniscus in her knee. In addition, she said, "I walk a lot. I love my walks with my little dog."

Mary said she starts the day with a low-fat breakfast bar. For lunch, the salad bar with fat-free dressings at local restaurants or her own kitchen have replaced Long John Silver's. And for dinner, "It's baked barbecue chicken, baked or broiled fish, and occasionally turkey breast, and once every other month maybe a boneless pork chop. Lots of baked potatoes with fat-free butter and fat-free sour cream, too.

She admitted she still has weight to lose, but who doesn't?

"I can honestly say I cook the same meals I did before, I've just changed ingredients. Meat loaf now consists of soy meat, mixed with two Healthy Choice Italian sausage links that have been zapped in the microwave and ground up. All other ingredients are the same, but I use Egg Beaters instead of real eggs. I also top it with salsa, for added zest. Lasagna, just change ingredients. There is not one recipe you can't change. Some just might take a little longer that's all."

"I have completely changed all my eating habits. If a product has more than four milligrams of cholesterol, I put it back on the shelf and walk away. [I] have really learned to cook differently, and use many products I never thought about before. It's fun, and challenging. . . . It just takes a little thought. If you make it fun, you will and can stay with it; if you make it a chore and complain, you will never stay with it."

"When I was in cardiac rehab, the nurse in charge was telling us one day that we could have things that weren't heart-healthy three or four times a year. I thought, 'Gee this isn't going to be too bad at all.'

"Anyway, one guy in the class decided he'd rather be dead than eat low fat, and went home and bought real bacon and butter, etc. He died three months later. That was hard for me, because his passing didn't have to be that way, it was his choice. My rule of thumb is, if I pick up any product and if it has more than 3 percent or 4 percent fat per serving, I put it back on the shelf and find something else. I will not settle for more. Again, it's my life, and I want to be around for my grandkids."

Heart-attack survivors learn that when they change their lifestyles, they often lose old acquaintances. Much like the alcoholic who stops drinking and frequenting bars with other problem drinkers, they no longer have much in common with friends who insist on smoking, drinking heavily, and eating fatty food, and see little benefit in working out and getting healthy.

"I had three real good friends," Mary said. "One was afraid to be around me and informed me we couldn't be good friends any more. The other two were afraid to be with or around me in case I had another heart attack. They wouldn't even come to see me for that fear. Needless to say, I soon gave up on them, and never answered their calls, and quit talking to them completely. I became really upset, too."

Losing friends helped Mary stop depending on them to get around and was an additional motivation to get her own driver's license. A stress-management class that was part of her cardiac rehab also helped her end her dependency on others. "I still use the techniques I learned there every day in my life. I would recommend this to everyone, not just heart patients. Learn and take time to relax each and every day. Do something just for you. You only live once, and you are worth it."

Mary's mother is still around. "My mother is still here. She had Paget's disease and can't get around real good. She's eighty-three, and writes down every time someone calls her, and the entire conversation. When you call her she then reads the entire list to you from the time you called last to present, then when she's done starts all over again."

Every year, on the anniversary of her heart attack, Mary sends her surgeon a thank-you note. "I'm thanking him, and letting him know I'm still here. It's been fifteen years since my surgery. I haven't had anything else done, and don't take medications that I didn't take when I first came home. That in itself is truly amazing."

Mary said that her latest lab work showed her cholesterol level was 120. Most doctors say the goal is to keep the number below 200. And she said her last nuclear stress test, which detects clogged arteries, "showed no real blockages in and around my heart except a small area about . . . the size of a small pea.

"Yeah, heart disease is reversible."

Chapter 9:   Morris Ginsberg

Morris Ginsberg likes to sit with his feet up in a reclining chair in his apartment thirty-seven floors above the Hudson River. Most of Manhattan is heading to work, but Morris, sixty-three, is working from home. That means that instead of a banker's blue pin-stripe business suit, this recovering heart patient is dressed in an off-white, zipper-front sweatshirt with a hood, blue sweatpants, a navy blue turtleneck and slippers. Morris's hair, straight and white, is combed back. A short, white beard covers his rounded face.

It's a clear day, and the view from the wide windows of his downtown New York apartment makes you feel like you're floating in the sky. Far below, straight down, are the churning waters of the cold Hudson, where US Airways pilot Chesley "Sully" Sullenberger ditched his plane in 2009, saving all 155 people onboard after the aircraft had been disabled by birds shortly after takeoff.

"There's the Goldman Sachs building," Morris said, pointing to a forty-two-floor, glass-wrapped tower. "And there's the Statue of Liberty."

This is downtown Manhattan—way downtown, in the financial district, across the street of the hole in the ground where the Twin Towers of the World Trade Center once stood. "I heard the second plane come in," said Morris, who was still home when United Airlines Flight 175 screeched past his window before plowing into the South Tower of the trade center. "The engines were roaring."

Morris lives alone in a one-bedroom unit. Oriental rugs cover the floors, Japanese fans adorn the walls, a grand piano sits in the center of the living room, and not far from that is Morris's desk, where he sits before a wide computer monitor.

It's Christmas Eve, and his monitor is flashing. That's because Morris is a financial trader, and on his screen are five or six windows full of flashing stock symbols in yellow, green, blue, and white. "Here's the S&P 500," he said, pointing to the symbol "SPX." "And that's Chevron. And this is Exxon."

For the past thirty years, he has needed to be near his work—Wall Street, where he buys and sells stocks. And it nearly helped kill him—the money and the lifestyle it afforded. Morris worked the hectic, high-stress floor of the American Stock Exchange, where he hurried about as an options trader. It was, at times, beyond intense. But it was well worth it, Morris thought, then and now.

He earned more money in a day than most Americans made in a year. The fringe benefits were incredible, he thought: women, booze and cigarettes, travel, and drugs in places where New York's finest would never come looking.

But eventually there was heart disease, which caused Morris's personal, self-centered partying to plummet like the Dow Jones Industrial Average on Black Monday.

On Wall Street, when someone has been whipped by the market, burned out by the stress, ruined financially, they call him a "broken man." Today Morris might still be seen as a broken man, but it wasn't the market that whipped him. It was his inability to cope with cardiovascular disease, despite all his money and some of the best medical care in the world available to him within walking distance of his New York apartment building.

He still carries the resentment that he, of all people, could be struck by a bad heart. It just wasn't fair. "My sense of self is diminished," he said. "You feel that you're not part of the world anymore."

Morris isn't his real name. He wouldn't allow me to use it for fear others from his past might read this book and find out about his decline. "I have lost everything I knew: my energy, love of life, rich foods, the man I was," he complained.

The world Morris built for himself was at odds with what it could have been, because he came from a strict, ultra-Orthodox Jewish household. His parents were from Poland, where they met before World War II and had Morris's brother, who is now dead. During the war, Morris's brother was sent to live with a Christian family, and his parents were imprisoned in Nazi concentration camps. They survived the ordeal and reunited after the war in Landsberg, Germany, the same town where Adolf Hitler wrote his autobiography, *Mein Kampf*. Landsberg is where Morris was born.

During and after the war, many Jews were trying to escape Europe.

"Some had to go to Australia, some to Canada. Some went to Argentina," Morris said. "They were all over."

Morris's family was granted access to the United States and in 1949 booked passage on a ship bound for Boston. From there they moved to New York, where they started a new life on the Upper West Side, on the corner of Amsterdam Avenue and Eighty-fourth Street. The Jewish community in New York was tight-knit. "Everybody knew everybody," Morris said. "Everybody had the same story: concentration camp, people who died. You heard this all the time."

Morris's parents worked at a garment factory, but they hated it and one day asked their rabbi to suggest another line of work. "The Jews need kosher fish," the rabbi replied.

"My father borrowed two thousand dollars—one hundred dollars from twenty people," Morris said, "and opened up a kosher fish store on Amsterdam Avenue and Eighty-sixth Street."

The place was called Belnord's Fish Company, and it was located in the ground floor of the Belnord Building, a rodent-infested apartment building occupying an entire city block. All types of Jews shopped at Belnord's.

"You'd see polished people who could barely speak English, but they were doing very well in the garment center. They'd come in with big jewelry and all," Morris said. "But you also had the Hasidic people."

In addition to selling fresh fish at Belnord's, Morris's mother began selling her homemade gefilte fish, a traditional Jewish patty made of a mixture of whitefish, eggs, carrots, and onions. Her gefilte fish was a hit with New York Jews, who were soon coming to Belnord's from all over the city. More than anything, it was that gefilte fish that brought the family success.

"What brought us into the middle class was that my mother started cooking gefilte fish," Morris said. "When it came to the holidays, every Jew in Manhattan had to have my mother's gefilte fish. There would be lines of cars."

The ultra-Orthodox form of Judaism that Morris's parents practiced made for a strict upbringing. Morris wasn't allowed to read magazines, watch movies, or experience much else of the fun that New York offered. And in his teenage years, he was forbidden from speaking to girls.

Morris's father put him on track for a traditional Jewish education, expecting his son would eventually become a rabbi. To that end, Morris was enrolled at the Yeshiva day school, a Jewish school located on the Lower East Side. "Getting there was a pain: it took about an hour by train and bus. Also, the school was rigorous—classes started at 9 in the morning and lasted until 6 p.m." It all made for a long day. And at the end of the day, he had to face his father. "My father used to beat the shit out of me if I didn't know things," Morris said.

Morris found the lifestyle imposed on him to be stifling. "It wasn't about being a Jew. It was a sin to do this, a sin to do that."

Ironically, it was the fish store that opened Morris's eyes to the world outside of Jewish Orthodoxy. "People would come in with mink coats," he said. And once, when Morris was about eight, a customer asked him if he wanted to ride in a Rolls Royce. Morris remembers how quiet the inside of the car was, even with the engine running. "You can only hear the clock," the man said. Morris couldn't even hear that.

"As a kid, you're like, 'Wow,'" he said.

He was equally impressed with the important people who passed through the fish market. "I remember when President Eisenhower used to come to Barney Greengrass, which is a smoked-fish house right across the street. You'd see his old Cadillac with the curved tail." Isaac Singer, the Jewish novelist, and Zero Mostel, the legendary stage actor and star of *Fiddler on the Roof*, frequented Belnord's.

"I heard *Fiddler on the Roof* in the fish store," Morris said. "[Mostel] and my father would argue about how you are supposed to sing [the] 'ay, yuy, yuy, yuy, yuy, yuy' [from *Fiddler*. They would be] screaming to each other in Yiddish."

Morris was a delivery boy for the fish store. His pedaling around Manhattan delivering fish helped open his eyes to the outside world. "What that bike did for me was give me freedom of Manhattan," Morris said. "I took that bike everywhere. That bike showed me the world."

Soon, Morris began to rebel against his strict upbringing. He started reading *Life* magazine, and whenever he could, he escaped from home to the exciting streets of New York. A favorite hangout was Forty-second Street. "I used to play hooky to see four or five movies a day," Morris said. "I remember the first time I saw *Some Like It Hot* on Forty-second Street with Marilyn Monroe. I was thirteen."

Morris had never a seen a woman like Marilyn Monroe. "Is there a human being that looks like that?" he asked himself. "I couldn't breathe. Nobody that I knew looked like that."

The movies and his other experiences on the streets of New York changed Morris. "That made me say, 'Oh, no, no, no.' I couldn't believe it."

From those films, Morris discovered that he liked women who were "cute, smiley, bubbly." To him, that type of woman was a *shiksa*, the Yiddish word for a non-Jewish female. "It was the *shiksa*—the non-Jewish girls—who always turned me on," he said. "The Jewish girls seemed like too close to family, and I never had any sexual interest in them."

His father was determined to keep his son grounded. "What he once did . . . was he took away my shoes so I couldn't get out of the house," said Morris, who was fifteen at the time. "And he shaved my head right down the middle so I looked like a fool. And he said to me, 'That's what they used to do in concentration camp.'"

It was so bad that at times, Morris said, he considered suicide. "I always thought I was going to get suicidal. I remember taking the train one day and thinking of jumping off the tracks if I didn't get out of the house."

Finally, at sixteen, Morris left the house for good. "That's it; I just can't be home anymore," he told himself. From that moment on, Morris was in charge—of where he would live, whom he would date, what he would eat, and how he would take care of himself. His father's beatings "forced me to leave home and become somebody else," he said. "I had enough of being told what to do."

That was the end of Morris's relationship with his parents. If either has had health issues in their old age, Morris can't say. He never contacted them about his own heart condition.

In the beginning, he said, he was "living here, living there."

"I was living with friends, on couches, [in] dorms. I just couldn't be with my parents."

He took some classes at Columbia University and the Juilliard School in classical music, which had always been Morris's passion. At night he drove a taxi, tended bar, and played classical music at local concert halls. Drugs and rock and roll were also a big part of his lifestyle.

"I knew Jimmy Hendricks, Jim Morrison. I knew them when they were just regular guys," Morris said. "Richard Pryor and I went to see James Bond movies together."

It was a life about as far from Orthodox Judaism as possible. "I evolved into somebody else," Morris said. "Completely at odds with my background. Completely."

Morris was sleeping around a lot, too, and in his mid-twenties, in 1970 or 1971, he got a girl—a non-Jewish girl—pregnant. "The next thing I know, I'm a dad."

Morris married the mother of his child. "I took on the moral responsibility," he said. "I shouldn't have married her. It was a big mistake. We fought all the time. It was awful." The couple divorced after seven years.

For most of his twenties, Morris floated from job to job. Then, when he was thirty, some friends called to talk to him about a job. It was 1976. "We're doing some things down here on Wall Street," they told Morris. "Why don't you come down and take a look. Maybe you can get into it."

Morris liked what he saw and took a job with a small trading firm. He moved around a few times before settling as an options trader on the floor of the American Stock Exchange, just off Wall Street.

What Wall Street brought Morris was a high-speed, high-stakes life; a life free of want; a life of excess; a life of everything forbidden to an Orthodox Jew. It was also an unsustainable life, and one that would have its consequences.

Almost every workday started the same. Morris would rise early, read all the newspapers he could find, and do a few simple exercises. He'd then leave for the stock exchange, arriving about nine fifteen.

Unlike today, when computers do much of the actual trading, the floor (also known as the "pit") of the American Stock Exchange in the 1970s and 1980s was often a frenetic mass of aggressive traders (mostly men) in pin-stripe suits, crammed together, arms flailing as they shouted buy and sell orders to clerks on the balcony above.

"How you making the Beamer," one guy might shout, referring to IBM.

"Five to a quarter . . . Five! A thousand up," someone might reply.

"What's the market now?"

"Five to three eighths."

"How many?"

"A thousand up."

This type of high-intensity, back-and-forth trading might continue for hours, or perhaps all day, depending on the movement of the market.

"It's stressful work, but some people are suited for stress," Morris said. And those who aren't suited for the stress?

Morris said you can pick them out of crowd. They get a "pale color in the face," he said, and they look like someone who was knocked out after a fight. After a couple of months they burn out and have to leave.

Not every moment on the stock exchange was so frantic, however. There were times, Morris said, when the market slowed and things were quiet. During those times, the guys found creative ways to have fun. Once, they dared a colleague to eat a cockroach from the trading floor. Another time they bet a fellow he couldn't eat 120 chicken wings in one sitting.

But Morris's favorite was the time someone tried to drink a gallon of water in five minutes. All the traders gathered to watch. "There's four hundred people in a crowd," Morris said. "People betting on him. People betting against him. Side bets. Serious money was going around."

The fellow managed to down three quarts, but the fourth was giving him trouble. "He's gonna blow!" someone yelled—and an instant later he vomited all over the floor.

At any moment, such pranks could be interrupted by a change in the market. "There'd be nothing going on," Morris said. "Then all of a sudden, you'd hear a roar. And you'd see people screaming and yelling at each other."

Working on Wall Street suited Morris well. It was *so* New York and *so* high-paced, and anything a man wanted was at his fingertips. To convey an image of New York in the 1980s, before the Internet bubble burst, Morris quotes Edgar Allan Poe's poem *To Helen*: "...the glory that was Greece / And the grandeur that was Rome."

On most days, the party started on the bottom floor of the American Stock Exchange building in Harry's, a legendary bar with a white awning. Harry's had a few locations, the most popular being at Hanover Square, where all the Wall Streeters went. But the location at the American Stock Exchange was popular, too. It was here that the traders often gathered at about 4:30 p.m., just after the market closed. Morris's drink was Remy Martin cognac, and he could put quite a few of them back.

After a number of cognacs at Harry's, the guys might take a limousine to a fancy restaurant: maybe Peter Luger Steak House in Williamsburg, the Four Seasons, or an expensive French restaurant.

The words "heart-healthy" weren't in anybody's vocabulary. "I'd eat anything I wanted," Morris said. "I'd have steaks. Then I'd have desserts." And with dinner there would be more drinks. "I would have a bottle of wine and four or five cognacs."

From there they might hit a strip club, or a massage parlor, or just another bar to keep drinking, and this was most weeknights. One can only imagine what the weekends would bring.

In 1980, Morris got married again, this time to a ballerina from Ohio. "She was the most beautiful human being I ever saw," he said. "She was eighteen, and I was thirty-three."

But not even marriage could slow Morris's lifestyle. In the early 1980s, cocaine appeared on the party scene. "I did a lot of drugs," Morris said. "Mostly cocaine." The coke kept the party going until all hours of the night. Often, Morris would get so wound up he'd need sleeping pills to help him get a few hours of restless sleep before waking up for work the next day. "You would come into work with a hangover," he said.

Morris was also a heavy smoker, going through about a pack every day. "It's a good, strong cigarette," he said of his brand, Winston. "It's got high nicotine content. I used to wake up and have a cigarette and play Beethoven."

Sleeping around was also one of Morris's weaknesses, and again, not even marriage stopped him. "It dominated my life in my twenties and thirties," he said of casual sex. "I was in heaven. I loved it. It was just great, and I knew at the time it was great."

Many financial traders shared a similar lifestyle. "Guys would go do their own thing," he said. "Some guys would go to Atlantic City. Some guys would go to Vegas. Some guys went straight to whorehouses. They'd make a phone call before arriving to find out what girls were available: 'We're coming over, close the place down.' You'd tell them exactly what you wanted, and it was provided."

"It was the lifestyle," Morris said of those years. "It was enough cake to kill a horse."

He never felt an ounce of guilt, or that it could end with grave consequences, like an overdose, or a car crash, or a drug-induced heart attack. "I wasn't guilt-bound by anything. That's how I was living my life at the time."

When he wasn't partying, evenings were spent playing racquetball with co-workers on the courts at the World Trade Center. He also rode his bike on weekends, and there was the occasional walk. "I felt that I was doing enough physical exercise that I didn't feel harmed by it. And I was enjoying myself."

Morris kept up his excessive lifestyle for nearly thirty years, and seldom during that period did he see a doctor. Sometimes, someone would ask him who his primary-care physician was. Morris could never understand why anyone would regularly visit a doctor. "What, are you kidding me?" he said. "Why? Are they going to give me good news?"

Only once, at the urging of a friend, did he get a physical examination. "We went and we had a complete checkup," Morris said. "The next thing I knew, [the doctor] tells me twelve things I shouldn't do and gives me four pills to take."

Morris took the pills, but immediately he felt side effects. "I'm peeing all day long, and my stomach is upset," he said. Morris called the doctor and asked him what do to. "Keep on taking it," the doctor said. "It's good for you." Morris didn't like that answer. "Get out of here," he told the doctor. "Forget it. Thank you. Goodbye."

One of Morris's greatest pleasures was escaping to the Caribbean when things started to get too stressful at work. "When I thought I was burning out, when I thought I was making mistakes, I would immediately go to the Caribbean somewhere."

Vacations far from Wall Street were necessary for Morris to clear his mind. "You have no idea how important it is to get out of town, how wonderful it is to forget, to resurrect yourself."

He liked going to the all-inclusive resorts of Club Med, like the ones in the Virgin Islands, Turks and Caicos, and Columbus Island, in the Bahamas Out Islands. When he'd go to Club Med, Morris said, he would sometimes swim miles offshore, right out into the middle of the Caribbean Sea, so far from shore he couldn't see land. For him it was a thrill, something to do. "You do it because it's there, and you have to do it. You're mesmerized. I get a big kick out of being alone in open water." The water is deep enough to drown, but even two miles out, the depth is only about twenty feet.

Morris said he'd been to the islands thirty or forty times over the years, sometimes going three or four times a year. "If I wanted to hop on an airplane, I did," he said.

Though he was married to his second wife during this period, she seldom joined him on vacation. Sometimes, he said, people would ask him why he went alone. "To have a good time," he'd answer. That's because to Morris, having a good time means answering to no one, having the freedom to do as he pleases.

The few times he took his wife to the Bahamas, they argued. "No, I don't want to do this," she would say. Or, "No, you can't wear that." He felt he couldn't do as he pleased. "It's not me at all," he said.

Morris ended up divorcing his second wife in 1987, after seven years of marriage.

Though there were up and down years in the stock market, Morris said he did well. "I've had pretty big moments. On a good day, you might clear fifty, sixty, or one-hundred-thousand dollars for the firm," Morris said. "But you have bad days, too."

He continued working on Wall Street until 2002. That's when he took a retirement package from Goldman Sachs, the company that acquired his previous employer. Morris retired partly because he didn't like the culture at Goldman. "Guys worked from 6 in the morning to 9 o'clock at night," he explained. "And they were the most aggressive assholes you've ever met. The Goldman credo is, 'Let's put these animals together and watch them kill themselves. And whoever survives, we are going to make a partner.'"

The terrorist attacks of Sept. 11, 2001, also made him realize it was time for a change. "After 9/11, I said, 'That's it,'" Morris explained. "I took a retirement package and started traveling." For the next few years, he traveled the world: the Caribbean, Asia, the French and Italian Rivieras. "I had the energy to do it, and it was great," he said.

It had been a wild, high-intensity life, but in spring 2006, everything changed.

One morning during a walk near his apartment, Morris was having trouble catching his breath. Reluctantly, he went to a doctor, where he learned that in addition to the painful shingles he had been battling, he was experiencing severe angina pectoris.

It's not quite a full-blown heart attack, but angina is a symptom of coronary artery disease. It happens when an area of the heart muscle doesn't receive enough oxygenated blood, usually caused by atherosclerosis, a build-up of plaque in the arteries. Though angina is almost always a sign of coronary disease, it doesn't always precede a heart attack. In fact, many cases of angina can be treated with medication. Only serious cases require any type of surgery.

Morris's case, however, was severe—so dangerous the doctors couldn't treat it with stents or angioplasty. The only way they could treat Morris, they told him, was with triple-bypass surgery.

Morris was admitted to Downtown Hospital, and three days later he was moved uptown to New York University Hospital. While he waited, Morris learned another piece of disturbing news. In addition to his having angina, the doctor's discovered he was diabetic.

Diabetes is a metabolic disorder in which the body doesn't produce or doesn't properly use insulin, a hormone that converts sugar and starch into energy. Although the causes of diabetes are not fully known, it's clear that genetics, environmental factors, and lack of exercise play a role. According to the American Diabetes Association, about twenty-three million people in the United States, close to 8 percent of the population, have diabetes. Many of them are unaware they have it.

Although diabetes is dangerous by itself, the condition is often associated with other medical problems, including heart disease or stroke. In fact, about 65 percent of diabetes patients eventually die of heart disease or stroke, and with diabetes, heart attacks strike earlier in life and are more deadly.

If Morris knew one thing about diabetes, it was that having it would mean he'd need to change his diet. That's why he wouldn't accept the doctor's diagnosis.

"You have diabetes," the doctor said.

"No, I don't have diabetes," Morris replied.

"Yes, you do have diabetes."

"No, I *don't* have diabetes."

This went on and on between Morris and the doctors, but it was no use. Morris's diet needed to change immediately, and that meant right then and there, in the hospital. "Instead of eating like a normal patient, I was being fed like a diabetic," he said. "The food is just a dried piece of bread. It's just awful."

The food was the least of Morris's worries. Though the doctors assured him that bypass surgery was relatively routine, Morris was terrified he was about to die. "When somebody tells you they are going to open you up . . . it can kill you," he said. "Also, I don't know what they are going to find. They're going to open you up and go, 'Oh, my God, this guy's dead.'"

Part of his fear came from the fact that Morris doesn't consider himself to be a young man anymore; he says he feels old—even elderly—and that as such, he has less "life force." At sixty years old, Morris said, "you've lived a long time; you're tired; you've seen everything." Life at that age, he said, is so repetitive, so boring. "I've read this book before. I've seen this movie before. I've seen these people before. It becomes familiar."

Morris feels this way because he had so much energy before his heart problems; so much desire to live a full, active, aggressive, and spontaneous life. "You have much more desire to live when you are thirty than when you are sixty," he said.

During the five days Morris was hospitalized prior to surgery, he was preparing to die. "I was . . . calling everybody that I know and telling them goodbye. I thought this might be the end." To one friend, he said, "This is what a condemned person must feel like."

But it wasn't just death that Morris feared; it was, as it always had been with him, a fear of suffering pain. That fear goes way back to the beating he once suffered at his father's hand. "I told the surgeon, 'I don't want to come out of this halfway. If anything happens to me, I want to end it.'"

Morris also spoke to the anesthesiologist about the pain. He was afraid that all the drugs he'd taken in his life could alter the effectiveness of the anesthesia.

"Listen," he told the anesthesiologist, "make sure that I get a good dose, because I might have some kind of immunity."

"Have you ever taken any drugs," she asked him.

"Have I taken drugs? I grew up in the city," Morris responded.

"Well, which ones have you taken?"

"How much time have you got?" Morris said, chuckling. "I've done enough. I just don't want to be awake."

The nurse just laughed.

Despite his fear of death and concern about experiencing pain, Morris made peace with himself. "I had done everything I wanted to do," he said. "I didn't have anything open. I was very much at peace. I just didn't want to be in pain."

After five days in the hospital—the time required for the Plavix to exit his body—Morris underwent triple-bypass surgery. The procedure went fine, but when Morris awoke, sure enough, there was pain. "You're open," he said. "You are effectively open. Somebody broke your ribs to get in there. . . . I was in pain. Enormous pain."

Morris shared a room with a heart patient who was eighty years old and had just come out of his second bypass surgery. He seemed to be doing fine, even after his second surgery. *How could that be?* Morris wondered. *How could somebody go through that torture twice?* There was only one answer, Morris figured. "Some people are more suited for bypass than others," he decided.

During his recovery period in the hospital, friends came to wish him well and to cheer him up. "Morris, you look great!" his friends would say. Morris wanted to say, "Oh really? I feel like shit." Instead, his sarcasm kicked in. "Well, I guess heart disease suits me," he'd say.

Every morning in the hospital began the same way for Morris. Three doctors would come in while doing their rounds and stand before Morris's bed in a triangle. "The shortest, most aggressive one would be in the front," Morris said. Then the doctors would ask him how he was doing, and jot notes on their charts.

On the fifth or six day after surgery, the lead doctor told Morris, "You're leaving today."

Leaving? They must be kidding, Morris thought. He could barely move. He was bedridden, and the pain was still terrible. And at home he'd be all alone. They couldn't possibly expect him to leave today.

"I'm not ready to leave today," he shot back at the doctor. "I can't. Who's gonna take care of me? I can't take care of myself. How am I going to cook? How am I going to go from here to there?"

"I don't know," she replied, "But you are leaving today. You can't stay here."

Morris didn't like that answer, and he demanded to speak with the hospital's patient liaison. He knew that the hospital had an in-house cardiac-rehabilitation unit. Maybe he could check into that facility for a little longer.

Soon the liaison, "a nice old lady," entered Morris's room. "If you would have been over sixty-five, you automatically would have gone [to the rehab unit] because of Medicaid," she told him. "But not with United Healthcare," she said.

Morris wouldn't budge. "Well, I'm not ready," he told her defiantly.

"We'll see," the liaison responded.

A few hours later, Morris was officially discharged from the hospital. His son and daughter-in-law arrived to drive him home. "They kick you down the stairs," Morris said of being forced out.

He was in a foul mood, made worse by the jolting of the car over Manhattan's potholes as they sped downtown. "I remember every bump on the ride going home," he said. "I was in pain. Enormous pain."

The hospital liaison made sure Morris wasn't completely alone, arranging for a nurse to check on him at his apartment a few times every day. But even with that assistance, the first few days were brutal. "You just feel pain," Morris said. "Breathing was so hard. You're in shock. You are alone."

Accomplishing the regular, everyday things—like bathing—were most difficult for Morris. "You are scared to take a bath; you are scared to take a shower. I had to put in a pole along the shower so that I could hold on. I put in a chair in the bathtub."

He also had to adjust to a drawerful of drugs the doctors prescribed. "Here's a guy who never took any pills, and now I've got eight pills to take a day." His medications include diabetes drugs like Avandia and Glimepiride, heart drugs including Plavix, the cholesterol medication

Lipitor, aspirin, and a B12 vitamin. Morris also takes a medication that keeps his heart from beating more than 120 times per minute.

"So, here I am, drugging up again like in the '60s," he said.

In addition to those medications, Morris often also needs Percocet for back pain, which he is convinced was somehow exacerbated by the open-heart surgery. "Nobody is relating the two," he said, "But my sense is, bypass led to back problems."

Morris made it through the first few weeks after surgery, but things didn't improve as much as the doctors had said they would. "They lie to you," he said of his doctors. "They tell you, 'In three months you'd be doing this and doing that.'"

That wasn't the case for Morris. "Walking was difficult," he said. His center of gravity also feels off-kilter, which Morris also attributes to the surgery. And he still has pain in the spot where they cracked his ribs for the surgery. "The nerve endings never came together. Sure, they tell you the nerve endings will reconnect seamlessly, but they didn't. Touch me here," he said, pointing to the center of his chest, "and I'll jump."

Though it's been more than two years since surgery, Morris still lacks energy to do most of the things he once did. He can't exercise the way he used to—he gets short of breath easily. And because he gets so much less physical activity, the time leaves a void in his life. He has all this down time, with nothing to do.

Morris also recently started having knee problems, and he frequently gets strange pains across the front of his abdomen. Though many of his ailments are likely the result of aging, Morris can't help but think everything was made worse by his open-heart surgery.

Morris's life bears no resemblance to what it was when he was younger. Though he does daily exercises in his apartment, he can no longer bike, play racquetball, swim or take long walks. And as for his true passion, playing piano, he finds himself doing much less of it today. "I used to play piano for hours," he said. "Not anymore."

Morris also seldom takes last-minute jaunts to fancy, all-inclusive clubs in the Caribbean any more. "I used to walk fast and talk fast," he said of his youth. "But I never got that back."

Because of his heart disease and diabetes, Morris's diet has changed dramatically, too. His first cardiologist wouldn't let him eat anything good, he said. And because Morris was terrified of dropping dead, he followed the doctor's orders. "I was eating shit," he said. "Cardboard." Because of his diabetes, not even fruit was allowed.

Finally, Morris had a word with his doctor. "You mean to tell me I can't ever have a glass of wine or a piece of fruit again?" he asked.

"That's not what I said," the doctor replied, snidely. "Just not for the rest of your *natural* life."

He changed cardiologists.

Now Morris has a more-tolerable diet. In the morning he has toast with light cream cheese, or diet yogurt. Only once a week does he have eggs. Lunch is often as simple as soup and bread. For dinner, Morris often cooks flounder or shrimp, and he enjoys it with a glass of wine. After dinner, he'll drink two cognacs, and sometimes he'll treat himself to a piece of chocolate.

All that healthy eating, as well as his light exercises, have paid off: Morris's cholesterol, triglycerides, sugars, and hormone levels are where they should be. "My numbers have been great lately," he said.

For a year and a half after his surgery, Morris spent almost all his time at home. It was terribly lonely—even his friends stopped calling. "When you are in the hospital, everyone calls you. [And] the first week at home, they call you," Morris said. "Then, nobody wants to [speak with you]. . . . And if you do get a phone call, you're not getting it because somebody wants to speak with you. It's because [they] feel it's an obligation."

When friends did call, Morris found it tough to relate. "You can't speak to them on your terms, because my life has become circumscribed to my apartment and my pills," Morris said. "You are not part of life anymore."

All the isolation started to wear on Morris. He would stay home all day, sometimes not changing out of his underwear. "You feel like you're a burden to everybody," he said. "I started feeling sorry for myself."

At about that time, Morris decided he needed to get out of the house and start doing something productive again. So he phoned an old friend on Wall Street. "I'd like to come back to work," he said.

"Yeah, come on in," his friend said. "You're good."

Because he had been away from Wall Street for so long, Morris needed to retake the Series 7 Financial Certification Exam, which qualifies corporate-securities traders. He spent ten days with a study book, passed the exam with an 82 percent score, and returned to work as a proprietary trader, which means he trades securities with the firm's money for the purpose of making the firm a profit.

"It's keeping me alive," Morris said of his work. "It gives me something to do."

But the work doesn't come as easily as it once did. He doesn't have the concentration he had. And in his line of work, Morris said, "It's all about timing and concentration." Also, in the afternoon, right around 4 p.m., when the market often shows signs of life, Morris finds himself growing tired.

Morris doesn't work as hard as he used to, and often he works from his home office, where he was one day when I spoke to him. Sure, he's back at work, but he's still not the man he was, and that saddens him. "I miss the physical part of my life. Now it's basically a home life," he said.

Morris doesn't have much of a family life lately, though really, he never did. Not too long ago, his only brother died of diabetes. And both his parents have died, though he hadn't spoken to them in years anyway. Even Morris's relationship with his son, who is married and lives in the same apartment building, recently deteriorated. "I am having problems with my son," he said. "I don't know what happened . . . we were close." It turns out Morris resents the fact there are no grandchildren. "My sense is that if you are married for a while and you don't have kids, it's going to be a difficult marriage," Morris said. "They both never grew up."

When asked about his current social life, Morris emitted a shrieking laugh. "There is no lifestyle now," he cackled. "You go home, you make something to eat, you lie down and you take a nap. Then you get up, and you look at the computer to see what the world markets are doing, and then you either read or play the piano."

What makes it hard for Morris is that there is so much to miss. He longs for the fun he used to have—the parties, the travel, the excitement, and perhaps most of all, the women. He still only likes younger women, but at sixty-three, they aren't an option anymore. "If I go to bed, it's got to be with someone under thirty-five, or thirty-two," he said.

Sometimes Morris thinks it's not too late to return to being the man he was. "You tell yourself to go back to when you could pick up women," he said. But he realizes that will never happen now. "I consider myself elderly. I have to adjust, and I have to rationalize to myself."

One of the best ways to explain what he's lost and how he feels, Morris said, is to compare his situation with the life of a professional basketball player. "It's like Michael Jordon. Compare him now to what he was when he was a star. He's not the same anymore."

The emotional toll sickness and aging have taken on Morris have been accompanied by another stress, that of watching world financial markets collapse in the second half of 2008. Watching the decline of the markets and the collapse of some of the financial world's most iconic institutions—Bear Stearns, Lehman Brothers, Fannie Mae, AIG—left Morris feeling he lived in a world he didn't know. After all, much of his life is intertwined with institutions that are failing. "This, to me, was almost a sense that the world as I know it was disappearing," he said. "It's the worst movie ever."

When he was younger, Morris never let the market stress him out. "In the old days, I would have been more crass. I didn't take it personally. But this time, I think I am taking it more personally. Because of your age, you become more sensitive. It's a form of slow death. Like having your eyesight go. Like somebody taking bread off your table."

Sometimes, everything Morris has been through weighs heavily on him. "Suicide comes up," he said. "There are days like that. When you are in pain, and you have no grandkids, and it feels like there's no reason to go on. I don't want to die in pain."

Again, Morris compared his feelings to someone else: "When Hemmingway shot himself—I understand that. He wasn't the man he was before. He couldn't play the sports he used to, or make love all the women he once did. I understand that."

Still, despite the pain of watching the markets fail, the longing he feels for his younger years, and all the hurt and loss that heart disease have brought, Morris remains remarkably defiant and unapologetic.

"*C'est la vie*," he said.

He also realizes that his life could have turned out far different. And in that regard, even with all that he's lost, Morris feels lucky. "The world is a cruel place," he said. "I could have been born in Poland, in a concentration camp, like my parents."

He also has no regrets—not the women, not the drugs, not the failed marriages, not even his lost relationship with his parents. That's because for Morris, it's more important to have an intense and exciting life than to have a long life. "It's not about longevity. It's about quality," he said. "If you are going to have a wonderful and intense life, you are not thinking about the price. When you go out and you swim nine miles out into the ocean, there's a part of you that says, 'You can die.'"

"If I lived my life again, I'd do it the same way," Morris said. "If someone told me, 'It'll shorten your life,' I'd have said, 'Screw it!' It was a wonderful experience, and you knew it was wonderful."

Some of Morris's pleasures have endured, chief among them music. His favorites are the classics: Beethoven, Bach, Mozart, Chopin. Such music is a passion to him, a form of expression and beauty that's unmatched. "It's a higher revelation than philosophy," he said. "It's the highest revelation."

Morris also likes contemporary tunes. On that cold day in December he played some of his favorite artists. First, Linda Ronstadt, whose voice made Morris shut his eyes and smile. "There is no number two," he said of Ronstadt. Then Amy Winehouse, who is deep and full and rich with emotion, radiated through his apartment. "She's a real star," he said.

Just then, Morris looked at his watch. It was nearing 1 p.m., and today, the day before Christmas, that was the time the stock market closed.

The end of the trading day on the New York Stock Exchange is marked by the ringing of a bell. And though Morris is working from home today, he's not one to dispense with tradition. Resting on his desk is a small metal bell, the kind you see in cheap motels, with a handwritten sign reading "Ring for services."

Morris, watching the clock on his computer monitor and counting the seconds, extended his hand, palm down, and held it over the bell: *fifty-seven, fifty-eight, fifty-nine . . .*

His hand dropped, his eyes lit up, and a boyish smile spread over his face.

Ding, ding . . . da-ding.

Chapter 10: Neal Gregory

Neal Gregory leans back in a chair in the corner of the sitting room in his townhouse on Capitol Hill in Washington, D.C. It's mid-afternoon on a mild winter day, a Tuesday, and Neal is home early from work.

The sitting room is quiet, adorned with paintings of country scenes, and lit only by natural light streaming around the bare winter trees that line the street. Oriental carpets cover the hardwood floor, and bookshelves packed with a lifetime of reading line the back wall.

The place has a broken-in, comfortable feeling about it—like it's been a good home to the same people for a long time. It has. The house has seen Neal and his wife, Janice, through nearly forty years of life. It has seen them progress through careers on Capitol Hill. It has seen them raise three children. And it has seen them battle heart disease.

Neal was born in the Deep South city of Tupelo, Mississippi, on Aug. 1, 1936. Tupelo was a small town at the time—Neal said that when he was born, there were only about five thousand residents—and it was a pleasant place for a kid to grow up. It was a small town supported by agriculture—lots of cotton farming—and a mix of mills and manufacturing companies.

It was also a progressive city. It was the first to receive electricity from the Tennessee Valley Authority, a New Deal-era agency that provided electricity and other public works to the depressed Tennessee Valley, which stretches into Mississippi.

And though it's in the heart of the South, Tupelo was racially progressive. According to Neal, it was the first city to voluntarily desegregate its schools in the 1960s. Neal attended Tupelo High School, and during summers he worked at the Tupelo Journal, a newspaper with a circulation of thirty thousand that covered northeast Mississippi.

Neal's father was a salesman for a grocery wholesale company. He was also fond of fishing and hunting, two sports Neal never took up. Something else Neal never took up was smoking, though his father puffed King Edward cigars.

Neal's mother, like his aunts and many family friends, was a great Southern cook. The family ate lots of fried foods, and all the vegetables were cooked in pork fatback with a sliver of lean meat. "Everything was fried," Neal said. "Vegetables cooked with fatback. Biscuits and gravy. Lots of rich desserts." Though Neal was never seriously overweight, he was a little pudgy.

After high school came the University of Mississippi, where Neal earned degrees in political science and journalism. He then worked as a reporter in Memphis, and in 1963, Neal won a congressional fellowship that let him spend a year in Washington. There he worked as press secretary to U.S. Senator Albert Gore, Sr, of Tennessee, late father of the former vice president and Democratic presidential nominee.

A few days before Neal arrived, President John Kennedy was assassinated, and just after he got there, Kennedy's body was lying in state in the Capitol Rotunda. Neal wanted to be there, but he didn't have an access badge to get him into the rotunda. He got in by flashing his Senate gallery pass with an air of authority at a Marine guard. "When [Kennedy] was lying in state, I was there, right behind the family, just by showing a visitor's gallery pass," Neal said.

For the next few years, Neal held several jobs in Washington, first with the Department of Housing and Urban Development, later with the presidential campaign of Hubert Humphrey, who was then Lyndon Johnson's vice president.

"I think [I visited] twenty-seven states during that campaign. And you had the Vietnam War protests. . . . [It was a] very exciting time."

Neal wasn't fond of Humphrey's opponent in the 1968 race, Richard Nixon, and he vowed that if Nixon won, he would leave town. It wasn't an empty promise. When Humphrey lost, Neal took a job in Rome as a press agent for a movie-production company. But the job wasn't available for three months, so he bought a Pan Am around-the-world ticket. The ticket read, "Memphis to Memphis." It was good for one year.

Neal started his journey heading west, stopping in Mexico, Tahiti, New Zealand, Australia, Indonesia, Japan, India, and the Middle East. In three months he arrived in Rome.

The Italian production company had Neal writing news releases from the set of the Marlon Brando film *Queimada*, which was released in the U.S. under the title *Burn!* Neal joined the crew for the final six weeks of shooting in Marrakech, Morocco.

"I'd write such things as, 'Marlon Brando went scorpion hunting in the foothills of the Atlas Mountains, where he is on location filming the multimillion-dollar production *Queimada*,'" Neal said.

It was exciting to be around such an international star. "We had all the European press coming in," he said. "We had the paparazzi trying to get a picture of Brando without his girdle and without his wig.

Though Neal made good money during this time, he was soon ready to move on. After filming ended, he traveled to the Soviet Union with a group of Europeans and did some freelance writing along the way. On Oct. 1, 1969, under an early snowfall, the young man from Mississippi found himself at the Summer Palace of Peter the Great. That's when he realized that after nine months of travel, it was time to return home to Washington. Neal headed back and took a job as a political editor with a new publication, the weekly National Journal.

For one of his stories, Neal went to Texas to interview J.J. Pickle, a Democratic congressman. While there he met Janice, who was from Corpus Christi. In 1971 they were married, and in 1972 they had the first of their three children. That same year they moved from a one-bedroom apartment to their current townhouse on Capitol Hill.

Because the National Journal was relatively unknown, the staff was trying to increase sales to members of Congress. Neal moved to the marketing and sales department, where he worked a deal that allowed House members to charge the annual $450 subscription fee to their stationery accounts, something members could already do with Congressional Quarterly. Soon Neal had sold subscriptions to about three hundred members of the House, earning a commission on every deal.

Though it was a lucrative year, Neal didn't enjoy marketing and sales as much as editorial work. So he took a new job in public and political affairs with the American Federation of State, County and Municipal Employees. Later he became director of computer policy for the U.S. House of Representatives, and then took a job as vice president of government relations with Hill & Knowlton, a communications consulting firm.

Neal eventually left to start his own business, the Gregory Company, doing public relations work for such clients as the Australian government, an organization of electrical engineers, and the Elks.

In all those years, Neal was never very physically active. "Aside from working in a bunch of States as an advance man for Hubert Humphrey in the 1968 presidential campaign, every job I had held mainly involved my sitting at a desk," he said. "My on-the-job lifestyle is still pretty sedentary."

As for his diet, Neal had a taste for high-fat foods like pizza, hamburgers, and Krispy Kreme doughnuts.

He started not feeling himself in 1996, at age fifty-nine. That summer, he and Janice traveled to Rome, where they walked around the city. Neal noticed that he was getting tired easily, especially when walking up the hills of Rome. It wasn't that he was totally out of energy, but he was fatigued. "I just thought I was getting older," he said.

Later that summer, on the morning of July 17, Neal's health worsened. He felt a little pain in his chest, but it went away as quickly as it had come. Later in the day, however, while at his office near Union Station, the pain returned.

"I was sitting at my desk in my office on Capitol Hill, when I got a sharp pain in my chest that wouldn't go away," Neal said. "The cliché about an elephant sitting on my chest comes to mind." Neal got up, walked around and drank some water, but the pain wouldn't stop. He called Janice for advice on what to do.

Janice knew it could be a heart attack, but she had little faith in Washington's ambulance service. This was during the years when Marion Barry was mayor, a time when city services were deficient. So Janice told Neal to put down the phone—but not hang up—and ask the person in the office next door to drive him to the hospital.

That person rushed Neal to The George Washington University Hospital. Janice also left for the hospital's emergency room. She arrived first and started filling out paperwork. "When I got in and said my husband is coming in with chest pains, they flew into possible heart-attack mode," Janice said.

When Neal arrived, the doctors knew what was happening. He recalled the ER physician greeting him with "Mister Gregory, you are having a heart attack." Before that day, Neal had no reason to think he was at serious risk for heart disease. His cholesterol was in the normal range, he never smoked, and he wasn't overweight.

But there was a history of heart disease in Neal's family: his father had died of a heart attack at sixty-five. His father, however, had been a heavy smoker, a habit that surely contributed to his death.

As Neal processed what the doctor said, the staff took his vital signs and administered blood thinners and pain medication. Soon, Neal was stabilized. The next morning, doctors performed an angiogram, which showed four blockages in the arteries around Neal's heart. The only option was to operate. One of the doctors spoke to Janice about the surgery. He had a little model heart, and he showed her where the blockages were and how the doctors would fix them. He also told Janice that Neal was lucky: Dr. Benjamin Aaron would be performing the surgery.

"Who's Benjamin Aaron?" Janice asked.

The doctor explained that Aaron was not only head of cardiothoracic surgery at George Washington, he was also the surgeon who operated on President Ronald Reagan after the assassination attempt in 1981.

"That's really nice," Janice responded. "But bullets aren't our problem."

They both laughed.

Surgery was scheduled for July 23, five days after Neal was admitted to the hospital. Five days seemed like a long time, and Neal asked the doctors if he could go home.

Not a chance.

For the next five days, Neal was stuck in his hospital bed, contemplating his future—wondering if he had a future. Making matters worse was the fact that on July 17, the same day as Neal's heart attack, TWA Flight 800 exploded in midair and crashed into the Atlantic off Long Island, killing all 230 people on board. As a result, all that was on television was depressing news coverage.

Though it was a tough few days, Neal said he never felt fear. He was just concerned for his family, and how they would get by without him being around. Though Neal wondered if they could it make financially, he was comforted because Janice had a good job.

"Fear was the one thing I did not experience. I loved my wife and children, and, of course, I wanted to live," Neal said. "But I had made my peace with God and was totally adjusted to whatever fate awaited."

In those first few days, Janice didn't have time to be scared. Things were happening fast, and she was distracted. "You are just getting through it," she said. "You are trying to think about what you need to think about. There is really not a lot of time for emotion."

Janice received the support of friends and congregants from their Episcopal church, where they had been members for nearly thirty years. Such support is helpful to many families who deal with heart disease. "When something like this happens, and you do have a supporting community, they call, and send notes and cards," she said.

Particularly helpful was Janice's neighbor Virginia, who lent a hand with everything, including driving her to the hospital to visit Neal. "[Virginia] just moved in on me and took over organizing me for what I needed to do," Janice said.

As they approached the day of surgery, Janice felt as though life was on hold. Her father had also suffered a heart attack at fifty-nine, and he didn't survive. That was part of the reason Janice had insisted Neal rush to the hospital when he first mentioned chest pains. Unlike her father, Neal was doing well. But even given the state of modern medicine and science, there are no guarantees of surviving open-heart surgery.

The night before surgery was difficult for Neal, but not because he was scared. At 2 a.m., another patient was moved into his room, and the man wouldn't stop snoring. "I didn't get any sleep," Neal said.

When daylight arrived, the surgery was delayed because of an emergency with another patient. Neal didn't mind. "When you are in the cardiac ward, it's not so bad to have to wait, because it means somebody else is a lot worse off than you are. Sometime during the hours leading up to his surgery, Neal had a vision. There, across the room, was Jesus, sitting down, wearing a heavy beard and a white rob, just like the image of Jesus in many a Renaissance painting.

"In hindsight, I wonder why he looked just like he is depicted in all the famous religious paintings, so tranquil in his white robe, with a glowing face, long hair and a beard," Neal said. "I asked him if he was ready for me, and he replied—in perfect, unaccented English—'Not yet.'"

"I have no idea whether I was going under the ether, or if it was a dream," Neal later said. "I was not at all afraid. That was the key thing."

Finally, on the afternoon of July 23, Neal underwent quadruple bypass surgery. It ended about 6 p.m., and Dr. Aaron spoke with Janice.

"It was late when Aaron came back after the surgery, and he said it had gone well," Janice said. Dr. Aaron also mentioned that Janice was right that Neal was a bleeder. "I thought we were going to have a problem, but we were ready," he told her.

As he spoke, Aaron reminded Janice of an Olympic athlete. "It was like somebody who had just run a big race," she said. "He was done for the day, and had just enough energy for the report."

After the operation, Neal was taken to the recovery room. Suddenly he started hiccupping and couldn't stop, and each time it happened, the pain in his chest was terrible. None of the nurses could stop them either; because Neal had just had heart surgery, they couldn't try any of the usual, old-fashioned remedies, learned outside nursing school, like slipping a cold key down the back of Neal's shirt, or startling him.

Soon, eight doctors, including the head of cardiology, had gathered to solve the conundrum. They all stood outside Neal's room discussing a solution. Neal found it very ironic. Here he was, just through with heart surgery—nothing short of a miracle of modern medicine—and no one could solve the age-old problem of hiccups.

Finally, the doctors sedated Neal with a cocktail of drugs. And to ensure he was left undisturbed, the nurses blocked his hospital door with a sawhorse and a sign that read, "Do Not Disturb."

Neal spent five more days in the hospital before he was released July 29. By that time, he was dying to get out of the hospital and eager to shower. When he got home, that's the first thing he did. But the combination of the hot water and the physical effort of showering was almost more than Neal's weakened body could stand.

"I almost passed out in the shower," he said. "I just staggered back to the room."

Neal spent most of those first days at home between the bed and the couch. He also watched a lot of television. "I was really tired, weak. You sleep a lot. There are people calling, there's people coming by."

The community support continued; for two weeks, Janice didn't have to cook a thing because friends and neighbors brought food. "Someone was organizing our food," she said. "We didn't have to worry about eating."

"And she didn't have to go to the grocery store," Neal added.

More than anything, Janice was relieved that Neal was alive. "He survived the surgery. I wasn't thinking too far in advance."

The heart attack and open-heart surgery were a wakeup call for Neal, and he began changing his lifestyle soon after coming home. One of the things to change was his diet. Gone were the high-fat dishes they used to eat. Gone were the pizza, the hamburgers, and the Krispy Kremes.

Janice and Neal began cooking low-fat Southern dishes. With the help of one of their favorite magazines, *Eating Well*, they've learned a number of tricks to reduce fat and cholesterol from their cooking.

"They do makeovers," Janice said of the magazine. "Like a pound cake with a third of the fat and half the sugar."

"Some recipes call for three eggs," Neal added. "But you can use one egg and two egg whites. It has all kinds of adjustments like that."

Janice said most people cook with fat because it adds flavor, but she's learned to use spices instead to add taste. "If you use three or four spices in something, you don't need all that butter," she said.

They also eat lots of fresh or frozen vegetables, and Janice learned some tricks to make them more flavorful. "We'll take asparagus, and instead of putting butter on it, we mix up a little bit of olive oil and orange juice," she said. "And you can put margarine in peas instead of butter."

And instead of cooking green beans in fatback, Janice cooks them with onions, sugar, and a bit of oil. "It's great," she said.

Janice has even modified some of the old dishes Neal's mother used to cook, like cornbread. Instead of making the cornbread with bacon drippings, as the original recipe calls for, Janice uses canola oil. She also uses low-fat buttermilk and egg whites.

"You can eat healthy and still eat Southern," Neal said. "The taste is almost the same."

Neal and Janice now eat fish several times a week, too. But unlike in the old days, the fish is broiled or baked. "Before my surgery, I don't think I had ever eaten fish that wasn't fried," Neal said.

They also like lean pork, chicken, or turkey. "It's always the breast," Neal said. "It's never the dark meat."

Neal has learned to read labels, to see how much fat or cholesterol is in the food he and Janice eat. "And one makes a lot of interesting discoveries, such as the fact that plain old Hershey's chocolate syrup has no fat and no cholesterol," Neal said. Now one of his favorite foods is Edie's frozen yogurt topped with Hershey's syrup.

Neal doesn't completely avoid rich or high-fat foods. Dr. Aaron said it was fine to have ice cream and a piece of cake at a birthday party—but just one. And, the doctor told him, don't go to a birthday party every day, no matter how many children you have.

In addition to watching his diet, Neal takes Lipitor, which significantly reduced his cholesterol. "My cholesterol is so low that I feel no qualms if we're going out to dinner to have a creme brulee," he said. "But I don't do it all the time."

Besides changing his diet, six weeks after surgery Neal started a twelve-week cardiac-rehabilitation program. At first he was skeptical that he'd be able to do any exercise. He was just too weak, and he didn't want to stress his heart. "I didn't know if I could get on the treadmill or not."

When you're just recovering from surgery, Neal said, you're terrified that you might have another heart attack. Even a little indigestion can get you thinking you're having one. You also don't know if you'll ever be able to do anything physically active again. If you can get past those normal worries and push yourself, he said, you'll see that you're able to do much more than you think you can.

"You wonder if you will be able to get back to anything like a normal life, and I didn't know if I could even get on that treadmill or stationary bike. But you start slow and build up the heart, and you are wired up, with a nurse monitoring your activity."

After a few minutes on a treadmill the first day, Neal's confidence rose. "I can do this. This is fine," he thought to himself. After four minutes on the treadmill, the nurses stopped him. "No, I can keep going," Neal told them.

That first day at rehab gave Neal a tremendous boost of confidence; he conquered his fears and learned he was capable of much more.

Even Janice saw the change.

"He was a different person the first night after rehab," she said. "Mentally he changed that night."

As the days and weeks progressed, Neal slowly built more endurance and more strength. "They are rehabbing the heart steadily, and they monitor you all the time," he said. "By the end of the twelve-week program, hell, I was doing fifteen minutes at a fifteen-degree elevation without any problem at all."

After twelve weeks, he left rehab and joined a gym, where he continued his recovery, exercising three or four times a week. At about the same time, Janice suggested that Neal get a bike and start riding for exercise.

"I don't want to ride a bicycle," he told her. "That's work." Neal had thought of riding a bike as work ever since he'd been a newspaper delivery boy back in Tupelo. But Janice convinced him to give it a shot.

"I got hooked," he said. "There are great trails all around Washington."

In the next few years, Janice and Neal's love of biking grew. In 2001, the couple took an ambitious ride along a path from Pittsburgh to Washington. They made the trip, about 250 miles, in only eight days, staying at bed and breakfast inns along the way. They also biked three hundred miles in Denmark one year.

Neal's lifestyle change transformed his life. "I am in better shape than I was thirteen years ago when I had my surgery," he said. "It's clearly from diet and exercise."

He continues his regular medical checkups and frequent stress tests to ensure his heart stays healthy. One year the doctors found that one of his arteries was starting to close, so they inserted a stent. Other than that, he's had no other heart problems.

Now seventy-two, Neal still works at his public relations firm. Plans to retire in 2008 were put on hold because the falling stock market hit his retirement funds hard. When he's not in the office, Neal is often at The George Washington University Hospital. He's not there as a patient, but as a volunteer for Mended Hearts, a support group for heart patients. Neal is the local chapter president.

Neal makes his rounds at the hospital once a week, often on Tuesday, talking to patients on the cardiac floor. Mended Hearts doesn't give medical advice but helps by telling patients what to expect from surgery and recovery. It's an opportunity for patients to ask questions of someone who has been through the same thing. It's also a chance for Neal to encourage patients to enroll in cardiac rehab after surgery.

"We go by and assure them that they're not alone, and they have a lot of company, and I've been through it, and see if they have any questions about it," Neal said. "My key message is, 'You've got lots of company.'"

Neal thinks Mended Hearts is important because heart disease is so emotional. "So much of it is psychological. If you weren't worried, you wouldn't be human."

In addition to visiting patients in the hospital, Mended Hearts has monthly chapter meetings. Some funny stories have come out of those gatherings.

At one meeting, a particularly energetic survivor was telling the group how heart disease helped him change every aspect of his life for the better. "You've got to change your lifestyle," he told the group. "I changed my job. I even changed my wife."

Another time, one man told another, "Soon, you'll be able to have sex again."

"Really? Really? I can have sex," the man responded.

"Sure you can."

"You don't understand," the man replied. "I'm a monk."

But more than anything else, Mended Hearts lets Neal teach others what he learned from heart disease: that attitude is important, and a big part of recovery is psychological.

"It's all in the mind," he tells other patients.

Chapter 11: Barbara Robinson

She was abandoned with three small children. Barbara Robinson recalled that she had returned home from work to an empty apartment. Her husband had taken off and sold their furniture. All that was left for the twenty-four-year-old office assistant was to collapse in a heap on the barren floor until she could figure out her next move. There was no point in crying and feeling sorry for herself. She had been there before, deserted by a man who found marriage and parenting too big to handle.

They lived in Chillum, Maryland, just outside Washington, D.C., where Barbara had moved years before to find work and a better life than Elizabeth City, North Carolina, had offered.

Barbara had thought she hit bottom the day her husband walked out, but that certainty would be challenged years later by a sudden heart attack that she never saw coming.

She was born in Norfolk, Virginia, to a teen mother and a father barely into his twenties, and her parents never intended to marry. "She eventually left him and moved to Elizabeth City," Barbara said.

Barbara must have gotten her toughness from her mother, Katie, who could go toe to toe with any man. Katie never finished high school and had no job skills to speak of, but she was a survivor, like many black women in the South in the 1950s.

If you didn't get up and go to work in the fields or the factory, you at least had to hustle, and Katie could hustle with the best of them. Some people operated illegal lotteries, or "numbers" games. Others took in washing and ironing for their neighbors and white folks. Still others offered barbering and beauty services, like cutting, curling, and pressing hair, or shining shoes.

Katie became a bootlegger. She sold homemade whiskey that she bought wholesale from back alleys and farmhouses in five-gallon jugs, then resold from her home or through distributors. Katie's liquor was consumed on people's front porches, in their bedrooms, and in the after-hours juke joints where people partied on weekends till dawn.

Bootlegging was a good business but very competitive, and because it was a cash-only business, it was also very dangerous. "We were never robbed, 'cause people knew not to mess with her," Barbara said. Katie packed a pistol and knew how to use it. And word was she kept an arsenal of weapons in her home where the liquor was stored.

Barbara and her younger sister would often accompany Katie when she picked up and distributed her merchandise. This allowed Katie to keep watch over her girls, and it made the bootlegger less conspicuous as she traveled around with two small children in her car.

Barbara recalled one close call, a time when Katie should have ended up in jail. "I was about six or seven. My sister was two years younger. We were in the car with my mother, and she had the trunk full of bootleg whiskey."

A police car began tailing them after noticing the car traveling very slowly, with the rear of the old vehicle smoking and practically dragging the ground. It was being weighed down by the whiskey jugs, and the car was leaning to one side.

Katie was ordered to pull over. After the vehicle was searched, she was arrested and taken to the police station with her two small girls. It wasn't her first brush with the law, just the first with the children as "accomplices." Barbara recalled that a sympathetic judge let her off with a warning after hearing the poor bootlegger explain that she had been abandoned by an abusive husband and that selling the booze was her only way to get money to feed her girls. She promised to change her ways. She had no intention of doing so.

"We were really poor but never knew it," Barbara said. "We ate beans every night. One day after getting off the school bus, my sister started crying as we approached the house. And when I asked her what was wrong, she said she smelled beans cooking again, and she was tired of beans."

There were no doctors, no hospital visits to remember. "Black folk made do with what they had, whether it be medicine, or food from the hogs and chickens."

Health care began and ended with what Katie was able to provide for her children. Homemade remedies took care of colds, cuts, and fevers. A black child had to be practically unconscious to qualify for a trip to the emergency room.

It might sound strange, but people in those parts seemed just as concerned about how they would be treated after they died. All the old folks seemed to have small life-insurance policies. A white man would come around once a week collecting coins for those policies, which ensured there was money available for a proper burial when the policyholder passed away. The old folks didn't want to be a burden on their surviving kin, and they certainly didn't want their remains turned over to the city or county for a pauper's burial.

Barbara attended segregated schools. The teachers were good, but the books might have been missing pages. Instructors used their own money to buy supplies. The buildings could have used some paint and plaster. She attended P.W. Moore High School in the mid-1960s. She once recalled with pride that Jethro Pugh, a star football player at P.W. Moore, remains the town's most famous native. After graduating, Pugh starred on the nearby Elizabeth City State College team. He later became a standout defensive lineman for the Dallas Cowboys of the NFL.

Barbara graduated in 1968. Her class was the last segregated class at P.W. Moore. The following year, court-ordered integration forced black and white students to attend the same schools.

College wasn't an option for Barbara, even though blacks were able to enroll in colleges across the South in record numbers because of affirmative-action programs and easily available loans and grants. Affirmative action for Barbara meant getting a job. Her mother's bootlegging business didn't bring in enough to pay the bills. Besides, the girls were expected to make their own ways when they came of age.

Elizabeth City is sixty miles from the Norfolk-Virginia Beach area to the north, and sixty miles from the Outer Banks to the south. Barbara moved to Norfolk. There she had a job of little consequence, but she caught the eye of a "big city" young man who quickly and easily swept her off her feet.

Barbara was attractive: tall and thin, 5-foot-9 and a mere 120 pounds. She had medium-brown skin, long hair, and light-brown eyes that stopped a lot of men dead in their tracks. "They often asked if I was wearing color contacts."

She slept with the young man one time and got pregnant. Tommy was born. She also admitted, almost embarrassingly, that there was a second brief romance with another man and an immediate pregnancy that produced a second son, Andre. In both cases, the fathers made clear that marriage was not an option. Raising her two sons would be her responsibility and that of her mother. "You look back at your stupid mistakes, and you feel so bad," Barbara said.

A longtime girlfriend had already moved to Washington and had been encouraging Barbara to join her. They could split expenses. So, making the tough decision to leave Tommy with her mother in Elizabeth City, Barbara, then twenty years old, packed her few belongings and went to D.C. with Andre. They moved in with the girlfriend in a one-bedroom apartment over a liquor store at First Street and New York Avenue, in Northwest, a short distance from the U.S. Capitol.

The following year, in 1970, Barbara's younger sister followed her to Washington. It was often the case that young blacks migrating from the South would later send for family. Eventually, three women and a boy would be living in that one-bedroom apartment.

Barbara became a secretary, for Aetna Insurance Company in Washington. Her office was on Connecticut Avenue in Northwest, and she had to take two buses to get there. The trip took her through the nearby inner-city poor neighborhoods that she knew not to frequent after dark. In 1968, riots had destroyed much of U Street and the Fourteenth Street corridor, and very little had been rebuilt by the time Barbara arrived in town.

The trip to Aetna's office also took Barbara through some of the city's wealthy communities where embassies line the streets and high-rise apartment buildings have twenty-four-hour doormen and valet parking. That daily commute to work allowed the young mother from North Carolina to see some of the best and the worst of the nation's capital. It might have been about this time that Barbara decided she could make a life for herself and her two sons in the big city.

"I earned about eight thousand dollars a year writing insurance policies, and always sent money back home, if only four dollars or five dollars, on payday."

She returned to Elizabeth City often to see Tommy and her mother. But Barbara's future was still somewhere in D.C. One night, while at a club on Georgia Avenue, she met Calvin, a handsome, 6-foot, D.C. native, smooth, with a soft touch and a big-city rap.

"You never want to meet your husband in a nightclub," she said later.

Calvin had a good job as a bus driver for the transit system. They dated for two years and then decided to get married. The young couple moved into an apartment in Chillum. They had a daughter, Danielle. Calvin knew Barbara had two sons and seemed OK with that, she said. Tommy was brought up from North Carolina. The family was complete: Calvin, Barbara, Tommy, Andre, and Danielle.

Then one day, with the children in day care or at school, Barbara returned home from work to discover it was over. "My husband abandoned us. I came home from work, and he was gone, and he had sold all the furniture. The apartment was empty. By phone, he told me he no longer wanted to be raising somebody else's kids and said he sold the furniture to recover some of his money.

"I was devastated. I had rent to pay, food to buy. How was I going to do this?"

She recalled that one night, she had nothing left but a can of spaghetti to share with her children.

Rather than brood, Barbara decided to make some changes, beginning with herself. "I realized I had two young boys and a daughter who needed to count on me for a long time. So I gave up cigarettes, changed my diet from that good-old country food I knew, and started jogging. I knew my kids' future would be based on how well [and how long] I lived."

Besides quitting smoking, Barbara started walking every morning, then power-walking with weights, then running, first along Chillum and Riggs Roads, always careful to get back to the apartment before the children had to be awakened, fed, and dressed for school. That exercising may have helped save her life later, when a heart attack struck her without warning.

It seemed that along with the exercising came confidence, more self-esteem. "I came here from the South with a North Carolina accent. I was stupid like a lot of young girls, but I grew and learned."

Single-handedly, she raised her two sons and daughter. They moved from Chillum to Bladensburg, where she bought a house. All three children graduated from the local high school. Tommy started his own electrical company, and Danielle went to work for him. Andre worked for Sony Corporation and traveled to Sweden once a month on business. Each bought his or her own home, perhaps proving that children of struggling parents are often more self-sufficient and independent.

One morning in 1987, while Barbara, then thirty-seven, was doing her daily run on the Bladensburg High School track, she caught the attention of another runner who had been showing up regularly. Donald Robinson was also thirty-seven, easily 6 feet tall, a bit heavy at about 235 to 245 pounds. He was at the track with a buddy running three or four times a day while trying to recover from the breakup of his own fifteen-year marriage. He had a son and an adopted daughter.

"I was going through some changes," he said.

It was Donald's buddy who first tried to win Barbara's attention. She wasn't interested, and he eventually took the hint. Except for an occasional date here and there, Barbara said she was no longer looking for romance.

Donald was more her type. He worked for the federal government, investigating white-collar crime for a major agency. "He drove an old car, a light blue Chevrolet. The upholstery was all torn up," Barbara said. He was a Christian, and that was important for Barbara to point out, perhaps because the other men who had treated her badly did not attend church services on a regular basis.

Donald seemed genuinely interested in all that this woman had overcome in her life.

"I had given up on men," Barbara said. "I was through." She had become somewhat hardened by her disappointments and rejections from men. Now she was independent and a veteran of the big city, and there was no evidence of the naive country girl who'd left Elizabeth City,

North Carolina, nearly twenty years before. There was hardly even a Southern accent left.

"I liked her independence," Donald said. Barbara still had her cute face and her attractive figure, in large part because of her regular workouts. Donald laughed while admitting that Barbara's looks hadn't gone unnoticed. "She was a cross between Angela Basset and Halle Berry," he said.

They talked, went for breakfasts, then dinners. That went on for at least a year. Three or four times a week, they would meet at the Bladensburg track. Working out seemed like a struggle for Donald. "I liked sweets and always struggled with my weight," he said.

Barbara was more compulsive about her workouts. It had become good therapy—maybe even addictive, replacing the cigarettes.

The thought of seeing Barbara for workouts made it easier for Donald to get out of bed in Northeast D.C. at the crack of dawn. After his divorce, he had moved back into his mother and stepfather's home. "The more I got to know her, the more she reminded me of my own mother," said Donald, whose background was similar to Tommy's, Barbara's older son.

"I was the result of an affair my mother had," Donald said. "I stayed with my grandmother, Daisy Brody, in Raleigh, North Carolina, while my mother, Lizzy, went to D.C. to look for work. She was eighteen at the time and hadn't finished high school. I never knew my father." Lizzy told him his father was the son of a church deacon, but the family wanted no part of him. "He had three or four children by different women," Donald said.

Lizzy left a second son, David, in North Carolina. He was also born out of wedlock.

Eventually she met and married George Robinson in D.C. They sent for Donald, who was eleven or twelve at the time, and George adopted him and gave him the Robinson name. The family lived at Seventh and Kennedy Streets in Manor Park, a middle-class neighborhood. Donald went to Roosevelt High School, and then the University of the District of Columbia. He worked nights as a security guard to pay his way and eventually graduated with a business administration degree from American University in Washington. He then worked for the U.S.

Department of Housing and Urban Development, the Department of Energy, and finally the Federal Reserve as deputy inspector general.

Donald had been divorced and alone for about a year when he met Barbara. Before asking her to marry him, Donald met with her children. He knew they had good reason not to trust any man, especially the ones who showed an interest in their mother.

"I met with her children and told them I wasn't looking to replace their fathers or try and be their fathers. I told them I could be their friend, that I was going to ask their mother to marry me."

They married at a church they had discovered together, Rhema Christian Center. Barbara's children, Tommy, Andre, and Danielle, were in the wedding party, as where Donald's son and daughter. Barbara's mother was too ill back in Elizabeth City to make the trip to Washington, but her father was there.

Her prince charming had finally come along. But for Donald and Barbara Robinson, the fairy tale nearly ended suddenly and tragically a few years after their wedding.

If Barbara had any indications before then that she was a serious candidate for cardiovascular disease, she had ignored them, or they came disguised as some other discomfort. Women had little reason to suspect heart attacks back then. Their doctors were not even trained to look for such problems.

In May 2001, the couple had just returned from a vacation in St. Maarten. Barbara couldn't have been happier. She returned to work seemingly refreshed and worry free. "It was a Monday in May at four thirty in the afternoon when I had my heart attack," she said. "I was fifty-one years old. I'll never forget it."

She was working as an administrative assistant for a firm outside D.C. in Tysons Corner, Virginia. Still an avid runner and now just over 150 pounds, this African-American woman looked more like a college athlete than a candidate for cardiovascular disease.

"I was at work when the pain started," she said. "It felt like indigestion at first, and I kept hitting my chest, trying to knock away the pain. I decided to go to the ladies room that was in the corridor outside the office suite. Fortunately, there was a chair in the alcove on the way to the bathroom, because I started to feel faint. I slumped into the seat as my boss was coming by. She asked what was wrong. By then, my left arm was feeling numb, and my jaw seemed to lock."

Before Barbara could utter a sound—which would have been all she could do—her twisted body and pained facial expression signaled her boss all she needed to know.

"You're having a heart attack," she said, and rushed into the office to call 911 and Barbara's husband. She came back with a handful of aspirin for Barbara, which may have helped save her life by thinning the blood enough to allow some flow around the clot or clots that were blocking the flow to her heart.

"I knew she was right about the heart attack," Barbara said, "but I couldn't believe it. It didn't seem fair. I had my checkups with my doctor regularly, and my cholesterol was almost normal just two weeks before. How could we have missed this?"

An ambulance was on the scene in a short time. "The paramedics gave me nitroglycerine and took me to the hospital. I was feeling better when my husband arrived."

Donald had been at a going-away party for a co-worker when he got the call from his secretary, Carol. "She said, 'You gotta get out to Inova Fairfax Hospital. Barbara has had a heart attack.'"

That was how his secretary always talked to him. He didn't like a lot of wasted words. "Just tell me the problem, and I immediately go into resolution mode," he said.

But Donald couldn't believe the news he had just been given. Surely there had been a mistake, a misunderstanding, because his wife was super fit. "I'm the one more likely to have a heart attack, the one who is always stressed out," he said.

As deputy inspector general for the Federal Reserve, he always had to be right when he uncovered evidence that a co-worker had committed fraud and cooked the books. Someone was going to be fired or imprisoned as a result of his investigation. If he was ever wrong, he would have to answer ultimately to his boss, former Federal Reserve Chairman Alan Greenspan.

"If somebody had found me on the job suffering from a heart attack, I would have earned it," he said.

Donald rounded up Barbara's children and brought them to the hospital. Tommy, the oldest, was stoic, like Donald, not believing what he knew to be true. His mother could be dying, soon. Andre and Danielle simply fell apart. They wept openly and hid in each other's arms throughout their time in the waiting room. Barbara looked concerned, perhaps even afraid, when she was able to see her family.

"I hugged and kissed her, while thinking to myself, 'This can't be,'" Donald said. He and the children formed a circle around her bed and prayed: "Dear God we are coming to you asking you to protect Barbara and to help her and us to understand and accept your will."

Barbara later recalled that Donald "stayed until about midnight, but because we were told I'd have to stay in the ER overnight until a bed was available, he decided to go home."

"I decided everyone should go home, get some rest and let her rest, and we would return the next morning," Donald said.

"'Do what the nurses tell you,' he said, as he kissed my forehead goodbye," Barbara said.

"I had a male nurse who was so kind. 'Call me if you feel anything that worries you at all,' he told me. I was lying there, thinking about my own mortality, wondering if it could happen again, and worrying about my family. Then I remembered I had a couple of bills on my credit card I didn't want my husband to know about—silly little purchases us women all make. And then I started to feel just an inkling of discomfort in my chest. It didn't seem enough to worry anybody, but I had promised my husband."

"When I pushed the call bell, my nurse came right in and looked at the telemetry machine above my stretcher. He ran outside the curtain, and everything became a bit of a blur. I found out later I had a second heart attack, and that I had a stent put in my artery."

Later, her doctor, Joseph Robinson, told Barbara she was lucky she had taken up jogging and changed her diet. "He told me my heart muscle had grown stronger as a result, and having all that extra healthy muscle had saved my life."

Although she had changed her lifestyle, Barbara couldn't change her genes. Her mother had died of a burst aneurysm in a blood vessel in her brain, and her father had died of a heart attack.

Now Barbara has a medicine cabinet full of pills she must take every day as a preventive measure. There is a blood thinner, a beta blocker, a statin, aspirin, and a pill to keep her bladder empty and thus put less pressure on her lungs. She doesn't like having to take all that medicine, but she is thankful she hasn't suffered any of the possible negative side effects.

Donald said he had stayed calm during the entire ordeal because he was in denial and couldn't understand how someone so fit could suffer a heart attack. The gravity of what had happened didn't hit him until three weeks later.

He and Barbara went to Dr. Robinson's office, where they were shown charts and diagrams of her damaged heart. The doctor, never one to mince words, looked at the two of them and said, quite frankly, "I don't understand how this woman is even still alive after this kind of cardiovascular event."

Donald went back to his office at New York Avenue and Fifteenth Street, not far from the White House. "I closed my office door, put my head down on my desk, and cried like a baby," he said. "I realized how much my wife meant to me, how close I came to losing her, and what a gift God had just given us."

Barbara is still able to run three and four miles, four times a week. She is totally intimate with Donald, who had his own medical scare when he developed kidney disease and needed dialysis, then a transplant. "A donor came through, a twenty-three-year-old male from Texas, probably the victim of a traffic accident," Barbara said.

Donald added, "Her heart attack prepared us for my health crisis."

Barbara took off of work to care for her husband, just as he had taken six- weeks leave to help nurse his wife back to good health. Donald is now retired and "living the life," he said.

Barbara went through cardiac rehabilitation and was taught how to change her diet. "I eat yogurt and granola for breakfast, with maybe a handful of nuts. Almonds are my favorite. I always pack my lunch for work and include some fruit for a snack. Lunch is my main meal, and it is always a salad of some sort.

"Sometimes, I'll add tuna fish, skinless chicken breast, or lean roast beef. It's funny, even when we go out at work for lunch, I'll still always choose a salad. I've just gotten used to it, and you can eat a lot of vegetables without it mattering."

For supper, she said, she and Donald eat light, often cold cereal or even oatmeal.

They travel to North Carolina often to be with her siblings, cousins, nieces, and nephews in Elizabeth City. The family still owns the four-room house that Katie bought for her children with her bootleg profits. Katie's girls had indoor plumbing installed years ago. "We return home every chance we get, like most Southern people," Barbara said.

When they travel back south, Barbara and Donald do indulge in the deep-fried okra, chicken and potatoes, and fried cornbread they have mostly sworn off, but they do so in moderation. It's not every meal, every day.

Donald said they've learned not to sweat the small stuff, and neither seems resentful about their health experiences. Perhaps their early travails as children in North Carolina prepared them for what lie ahead. "I couldn't be angry, because I am still here. I was spared," Barbara said.

At her doctor's encouragement, Barbara always carries nitroglycerine with her, but, she said, "I've never had to take even one." Like a spare tire for a car, it's there if she ever needs it.

Barbara credits her recovery to her religious faith. "As a Christian, I believe God put us on this earth for a purpose. I guess my purpose hasn't been served yet. I think about God a lot when I jog. I love to be outside, early in the morning, surrounded by nature. God meant us to run on His earth outside, not on a treadmill watching TV."

"It's my time to myself, my time to think and to be grateful."

Barbara and Donald's blended family now includes six grandchildren. The couple moved from Bladensburg to Barbara's "dream house," surrounded by trees, in Glen Dale, Maryland.

Barbara said that before her heart attack, her obstetrician/gynecologist would measure her blood pressure and check her heart rate, but that there was never talk or concern about cardiovascular disease. Her family history should have been a red flag to her physician.

More American women are killed by cardiovascular disease than by breast cancer and all other diseases combined. Strokes are the third leading cause of death. African-American women like Barbara Robinson are 60 percent more likely to die of cardiovascular causes than white women, doctors say. Among African-American women, the poorer and less-educated are less likely to know the warning signs of cardiovascular disease, and far more likely to put off going to the hospital, cardiologists say.

Barbara wants more education to be available for all women, and better training for all their doctors, especially ob-gyns. She knows that she was more lucky than informed when her heart attack occurred.

"African-American women have taken their health too lightly," she said. "I have a new respect for heart attacks. It attacks you out of nowhere."

Chapter 12: Larry Harris

Larry Harris runs marathons. He likes to run ten-mile races and ten-kilometer races. Really, he just likes running, and he's been doing it most of his life, so he's good at it. Once Larry ran a marathon—over twenty-six miles—in two hours, forty-four minutes. That's an average speed of more than nine and a half miles per hour. It's also a feat that, not long ago, could have matched some Olympic times.

Larry always crossed the finish line at or near the front of the pack. "I'd finish in the top 2 percent," he said, matter-of-factly. Larry has a Type A personality, and his motto seems to be, "Why enter a race if you don't plan on winning?"

Larry, now fifty-four, has been running since he was a kid, when he used to compete in the eight-hundred-meter dash on his high school track team in Brooklyn, New York. Over the years he kept in top physical shape, running almost daily, studying martial arts, and lifting weights. At one point he could bench press three hundred pounds. Exercise always made him feel good. "I loved how energetic and healthy I felt as a result of rigorous exercise," he said.

Larry looks like the definition of "healthy": he's muscular and thin, with an estimated body-fat count of about 7 percent. He doesn't smoke, seldom drinks, and gets regular medical checkups. He was doing everything right and expecting a long, uneventful life. Sure, he had high cholesterol and high blood pressure, but he was exercising so much he didn't worry.

Then, in 2004, at age fifty, Larry learned that he had never been totally responsible for his good health, but that luck—as is often the case—was part of it. The marathon runner suffered a heart attack, one that would eventually require the insertion of nine stents.

"You could have been like Jim Fixx," Larry's doctor told him.

Most serious runners know about Fixx, a former smoker and overweight journalist who changed his life by running in the late 1960s. In addition to quitting smoking and dropping his extra weight, Fixx wrote the 1977 book *The Complete Book on Running*, and is credited with started a running revolution.

Though Fixx transformed his life through exercise, he wasn't as healthy as people thought. That's because he had a history of heart disease in his family, a risk factor that no amount of exercise can eliminate.

In 1984, at age fifty-two, Fixx dropped dead of a heart attack after jogging. The medical examiner in his home state of Vermont found that three of Fixx's coronary arteries were blocked by atherosclerosis, and that he had atherosclerotic damage to his aorta and to arteries in his legs.

Fixx's death, which was shocking because it happened to such a seemingly healthy person, sparked a debate on the benefits of exercise. Was it running that had killed Fixx? Some wondered. His death also highlighted the suddenness with which heart disease can strike. "The first symptom of heart disease is sometimes sudden death," Dr. Lawrence K. Altman wrote in *The New York Times* a few days after Fixx died.

Like Fixx, Larry Harris was plagued by his genes. All the running in the world could not have prevented Larry's heart attack. That's a tough pill for a marathon runner to swallow.

Larry's story began in the mid-1950s, in a row house in the Bushwick section of Brooklyn. It was in that working-class African-American and immigrant community a few miles southeast of Manhattan that Larry was raised by his mother and stepfather. "I lived in the 'hood," Larry said of Bushwick.

It would not have been a total surprise if Larry, like a lot of his friends, had gotten into trouble in this part of New York, but Larry stayed away from drugs and got decent grades in school. "I did enough to graduate," he said. "I was one of those guys that got by."

More than anything else—even more than his mother's hands-on discipline—athletics kept Larry on a straight and narrow course. He was crazy about sports, particularly track and field. "I was never the fastest guy," he said, "but I held my own."

In 1972, Larry graduated from high school and started classes at Hunter College, on Sixty-eighth Street in Midtown Manhattan. But school didn't seem all that important to Larry, and he dropped out. "I learned a lot," he said, "but I didn't take it serious." Looking back, Larry said, he thinks he wasn't mature enough for college.

But Larry wanted more from life than a college dropout could expect. "I didn't want just another job," he said. To find what life held for him, Larry needed to find himself first. Part of that meant meeting his father, a man he never knew.

At the time, Larry's father lived near Charlotte, North Carolina. So Larry headed south, stopping in at Highpoint to stay with relatives. From there he sent a letter to his father. "I wrote him. Let him know who I was."

That weekend, Larry's father drove to Highpoint.

"He asked me if I wanted to spend the weekend down there [in Gastonia] with him," Larry said. "And I said, 'Sure, let's go.'"

The car ride was tense.

"Where were you five years ago?" Larry's father asked his son.

"Where were you twenty years ago?" Larry shot back.

"What do I call you?" Larry asked.

"Pop," his father replied.

To Larry, "Pop" was his stepfather. "I can't call you that," Larry told his father. "The man I call 'Pop' is the guy that whooped my behind when I needed it."

Larry couldn't stay at his father's house that weekend—his wife didn't want to meet her stepson. But his father, an admitted Casanova, had a girlfriend, so Larry crashed at her place. The whole weekend, Larry saw little of his father. Once during the stay, Larry went to his father's house, only to be greeted by the barrel of a gun. "His wife wouldn't let me in," he said. "She pointed a gun at me . . . and said, 'He is not allowed in this house.'"

"The next time I saw him was when he was picking me up to take me home."

The weekend was a letdown. Larry's father was uneducated and a womanizer, and he held odd jobs. Worst of all, it was clear he didn't care about Larry.

But the trip wasn't a total loss, because it helped Larry appreciate his stepfather, Booker T. It also was a chance to meet new members of his extended family. More important, meeting his father taught Larry about himself. "It was a devastating weekend, but it helped me in life," Larry said. "I knew what I didn't want to do. I wanted to be a good father." The experience also taught Larry self-reliance. "What he taught me was, be independent," Larry said. "It taught me that you need to do things on your own."

With those lessons, Larry took a bold step: in 1976, he joined the Navy. It was something he had considered for a few years, but the weekend with his natural father pushed him to join.

Larry started at the bottom of the ladder in the Navy. "I was in communications, and because my grades were poor, I needed to earn my way to become an electronics technician," he said. "I needed to do all the dirty work."

It may have been dirty work, but it was important work, and Larry needed to be sharp. "You're on twenty-four-hour call out there on a ship all by yourself," he said. "Nobody else around."

From 1976 to 1979, Larry was stationed on the USS *Milwaukee*, an oil-replenishment ship. From 1980 to 1982, he served on the USS *Sides*, a guided-missile frigate. The Navy gave Larry what Hunter College didn't: education and discipline. "It did good for me," he said. "I grew up a bit. That's when I learned what education can do for you."

In addition to learning a trade, Larry saw the world in the Navy—visiting ports of call in places like Spain, Portugal, Italy, Yugoslavia, Germany, Scotland, Amsterdam, and Halifax. "I was on two ships, and I went halfway around the world," he said. This was during the Cold War, which made the experience more exciting. "You could see the Russian ships right next to you," Larry said.

Larry left the Navy in 1982, taking a civilian job with the Department of the Navy in Arlington, Virginia, as a naval electronics systems security engineer. In Washington, Larry met his wife, Paulette, a PhD of immunology and an immunology professor and researcher at Howard University. They married in 1985.

With Paulette's help, Larry went back to school, first to Prince George's Community College outside of Washington for an associate's degree, and then onto the University of Maryland, at College Park. "She helped me with school," Larry said. "She encouraged me to get the associate's degree and then the bachelor's. It wouldn't have happened if not for her. You need a good support system." Larry's degree was in technical management and information-systems management.

In 1989, the couple had twin daughters, Kimberly and Kristina; three years later, a third daughter, Alicia, was born.

Along the way to building a family, earning a degree, and starting a career, Larry managed to keep in top physical shape, running up to one hundred miles in a week. He also took classes in two styles of martial arts—one Korean, one Japanese—eventually earning a black belt in each. And he lifted weights, sometimes on his lunch break. "I could bench press three hundred" pounds, he said.

He was so strong he won the yearly push-up contest at work against the Marines. "You had to do 229 push-ups in 6 minutes," Larry said. "I am the only one that did it."

But Larry wasn't just interested in his own health. He wanted to help others, too. So Larry started working part-time at the National Capital YMCA, where he provided personal training, fitness assessments, and equipment orientations.

Learning this new field was hard work, and, like anyone might, Larry made mistakes. But the setbacks only drove him to work harder, to learn more. "Every time I messed up, I had to go back and read the books," he said. "I always had the books with me."

It was rewarding on so many levels. "I got more out of the National Capital Y than just being a trainer. It . . . encouraged me to strive higher."

To further his fitness education, Larry enrolled in professional-certification courses, eventually earning certifications in strength and conditioning, sports performance, and personal training. He also took a part-time position at the University of Maryland, Baltimore County, as assistant strength and conditioning coach.

Whatever Larry learned in class or on the field, he brought back to the YMCA to practice on his clients. "I used them as guinea pigs," he said. "It taught them *and* me. They loved it."

It was a good time; Larry was happy, dedicated to his work, and seemingly healthy.

Then, when Larry was fifty, he started feeling fatigued. He noticed his running stamina was down. But that didn't concern him, at least not at first. With work, studying, and martial arts, he was a busy man. He thought he was just pushing himself too hard.

Then Larry noticed something else: one time while jogging, he felt a burning in his chest. It was an odd feeling, but still, Larry didn't think it was a heart problem. "I wasn't overweight," he said. "I thought I was out of shape because I had been lifting weights. So, I kept going."

Larry finished the jog, but the burning in his chest remained. He said that one time at home, the pain was so severe it made him fall to his knees, "but it only lasted two minutes." Paulette insisted he see a doctor. Neither suspected that they should rush to the nearest emergency room.

Larry started with his primary-care physician, who referred him to Dr. Hector Collison, a cardiologist at the Washington Hospital Center in Washington, D.C. Dr. Collison gave him a battery of tests, including an electrocardiogram and a stress test.

Larry went back to work for a few days while waiting for the test results, and during that time, the pain worsened. His chest felt heavy, and once he was sent home from work after falling to his knees again in pain.

Finally, Larry went back to Dr. Collision for the test results. "You look pretty good," he told Larry. "But Doc," Larry responded, "my chest was tight."

Collison decided to do an immediate catheterization. He made an incision in Larry's thigh, injected dye into the artery, and took a look. He found that although Larry's heart was healthy and strong, his arteries were in dire shape. Three were clogged: one 90 percent, one 80 percent, and one 60 percent.

Larry was suffering a heart attack. "If they had closed, you'd be dead," Dr. Collison said.

A heart attack? *How could that be?* Larry wondered. He exercised every day. He saw the doctor regularly. It didn't make sense.

Larry was sent home with a nitroglycerin patch to keep his arteries open and an appointment for a stenting procedure in two weeks. When he told his friends what happened, they were as surprised as Larry.

"Everyone was shocked," he said. After all, this was the guy who won the push-up contest. "You?" they asked. "Heart disease?"

Larry did some research and learned something that made it all make sense: his father, the man he only met once so many years ago, had had open-heart surgery in his early sixties and died of a heart attack in 1995 at age sixty-four. Larry also learned that two of his siblings had died of coronary disease, and his maternal grandmother died of coronary artery disease. In addition, he discovered that his family history was filled with obese and diabetic relatives.

That was it, the missing link. Heart disease was in Larry's genes, and no amount of exercise could change it. Knowing that made Larry angry, particularly with his biological father. "The *son of a bitch* never did anything for me, but look what he did for me now," Larry said of his initial feeling. "I was angry at a dead man."

There were other emotions, too. "I felt like my body had betrayed me—my heart had betrayed me," he said. "There was a lot of self-doubt. I was totally depressed and scared."

Two weeks later, Dr. Collison opened Larry's arteries. He put two stents in one artery, two in another, and used angioplasty to open Larry's left circumflex, an artery that curves around the heart. The procedure was a success, and Larry was released from the hospital with suggestions for changing his lifestyle.

"I had to change my eating habits," he said. "I was eating a lot of shrimp, which has high cholesterol, and fried foods like chicken. So I cut all that out."

Larry also was advised to slow the pace of his life. He was doing too much, pushing himself too hard, the doctors said. Larry stopped practicing martial arts and cut back his hours coaching at the University of Maryland.

It didn't take long for Larry to return to his daily jogging routine. In 2005, however, he again noticed that five minutes into every run, he needed to stop and catch his breath before continuing. Also, about forty-five minutes into every run, he'd feel a slight burning in his chest. "It wasn't as bad as it was [before]," Larry said, "[but] I am thinking, 'What's going on here?'"

Larry went back to Dr. Collision on Friday night, Dec. 23, 2005. The doctor had a reputation for working incredibly long hours. There were scores of heart patients to see in D.C., Maryland, and Virginia.

That Friday night, Paulette was with the children in Bermuda, caring for her sick brother. Larry's mother had come from Brooklyn to be with him while his family was away.

Dr. Collison had decided to do a catheterization. He assured Larry, "If there is a problem, I'm gonna fix it." There was a problem: the balloon used in the angioplasty to open Larry's artery the year before had failed, and Larry's left circumflex was 99 percent closed. The doctor fixed it with five new stents, bringing the total number of stents in Larry's arteries to nine. Larry watched the procedure on a television monitor.

"It was thin," Larry said of his artery. "Then he put the stents in, and he said, 'Look at that nice blood flow.' I automatically felt a big difference. I really felt good, because I could feel the difference in breathing."

Larry didn't want to spend Christmas in the hospital; he wanted to spend it with his mother and sisters in New York. But having five stents implanted is a big deal, and Larry wasn't sure if he could make the trip.

"Can I drive to New York for Christmas?" Larry asked Dr. Collison.

"You're gonna be sore," he replied. "[But] yeah, as long as you get up every hour or so and walk around."

The next day, Christmas Eve, Larry was released, and at 10 p.m. he and his mother left for Brooklyn, stopping every hour so Larry could stretch. In about five hours, he was in his old hometown. "I spent Christmas and New Year's with my mom," Larry said. "It was the best Christmas present I ever had."

Larry spent the next few weeks recovering with his mother in Brooklyn. His wife, however, had to stay in Bermuda with the children. "They called everyday with my brother-in-law, who passed on. It was rough for them," Larry said.

Thought Larry felt physically better right after receiving the stents, the emotional wounds took longer to heal. His family helped him cope.

"She's a strong woman," Larry said of Paulette. "She handled everything around the house, and kept everybody calm. She said, 'Look, we are going to get through this.'"

Support also came from the many friends and clients that Larry worked with over the years as a trainer. "Clients and several members of the National Capital YMCA made sure I didn't get too depressed," he said. "Those guys at the Y kept me going. I would come in and work with these guys, and they made me keep a smile on my face when I was depressed."

Larry found that exercise also helped. "Exercise and working out helped me go through that," he said. "If you want to get over the mental part, working out helps in the long run."

His mood improved, and Larry learned to deal with the anger he felt toward his father. "I was angry at a dead man. A guy who has been dead for eleven years," Larry said. "I had to get down into my spiritual self. I had to forgive him so I could move on."

"I have forgiven him," Larry added. "It took a couple of years."

Larry's children, who were in their teens when he was sick, were also a big part of his recovery. They looked out for dad—tried to keep him calm and ensure that he ate the right foods. "You can't eat that!" they would tell him. It felt strange to be lectured by teenagers, but Larry knew it was for his own good. "I understand that they are looking out for me," he said. "They are very concerned, and I appreciate that."

The kids encouraged him, too. As Larry was recovering, they'd say, "You're looking good, Dad. When you gonna get back out there?"

Despite all the support, however, the fear of having another heart attack never disappeared. "I am scared. I think about it," Larry said. "When I ran this morning, I thought about it."

As it does for so many people, heart disease profoundly affected Larry's outlook on life. "Having this situation with my heart, you start thinking about things differently. You got to take life in perspective. I look at life differently. I stopped thinking more about myself. I appreciate life more now."

Larry said he was humbled by his heart attack. And he no longer takes his health for granted. "It is a gift to be as active as I am. It's all a gift."

Larry thinks that enjoying life is what's most important. "Any endeavor that I get into now, I try to make it fun," he said. "That's what you need to do. I don't care how hard a situation is, I try to make it fun."

Larry has a few regrets ("I could have been a better student," he said), but overall, he feels pretty good about his life. "I look back on my life and say, 'I did all right.' I still feel like a success. I reached most of my goals."

But there is at least one unfulfilled goal: Larry wants to get a master's degree in exercise physiology. In fall 2008, he applied to a program at Howard University. Going back to school is a big, scary step, however, and Larry has self-doubts. "I am very frightened," he said. "I haven't been to school in years."

The same people who helped him through his heart disease pushed Larry to pursue his dreams, including Paulette, who helped him with the school application. Larry's friends at the gym were also supportive. "These guys and others at the YMCA encouraged me . . . they got me going," he said.

Larry applied to Howard despite his fears because he realized that the risk was worth the reward. "I don't want to get to the point where I say, 'I should have,' or, 'I could have,'" Larry said. "If I don't make it, OK, at least I tried."

That way of thinking is new to Larry, a direct result of his struggle with heart disease. "Before, I said [to myself], 'I know I can do it,' [but] I didn't do it," Larry said. "Now, I am like, 'OK, let's give it a shot.'"

The hardest part of the school application was the personal statement, in which Larry had to explain his reason for applying. How to put so much on paper? "I don't know what to write," he said shortly before the application was due. Then it hit him. Larry had been through so much with heart disease, fought so hard, and learned so much. The experience made him want to learn more about the human body, and to help others deal with the same struggles.

Finally, he put pen to paper. "Having CAD [coronary artery disease] made me more interested in learning about the function of the human anatomy," he wrote. "[It] made me more aware, and more determined to make sure others understand health and fitness."

With his degree, Larry wants to help others, especially the African-American community, whose members, he said, are particularly affected by obesity, high blood pressure, diabetes, and heart disease. "Our community has a special challenge to appreciate the need to maintain a healthy weight and fitness lifestyle," he said. "I want to work to find more effective ways of translating awareness into motivation and action."

But it's about more than education. Heart disease taught Larry about resilience, personal strength, discipline, and dealing with the unexpected. "Even if you live a healthy lifestyle and do everything possible to take care of your body, there are things concerning the human body that you can't control," he said. Earning a Master of Science degree "will inspire others to strive for high goals, no matter what their age."

Later, he said, "Hey, it's never too late to attain goals."

But Larry has other priorities, among them spending time with three daughters who will soon be old enough to move out. Larry doesn't want to see them go. "I don't know what I am going to do when the kids move out," he said. "Kids—the only problem is that they grow up."

Because of his other priorities, there's no guarantee Larry will ever finish the master's program. But that's OK with him—he's proud of his accomplishments; the master's is a bonus. "I reached most of my goals," he said. "If I don't complete my master's, I don't feel like I am a failure, because I'm going to learn a lot there. And I will use that as an opportunity to let people know that you can achieve anything you want."

In the meantime, Larry continues working at the Department of the Navy and at the YMCA on weekends. And now, having been through heart disease, he doesn't let his clients give him any excuses. "I don't want to hear that," Larry tells them when they say he's pushing them too hard.

As for his own physical health, Larry is doing great. "Right now, I've got just as much energy as I had when I was thirty or forty years old," he said. "I feel good. I look great." And he exercises regularly. "Right now, I am running about fifty miles a week."

Larry is more vigilant about his body now. He also communicates how he feels to his wife and children. And if he ever feels burning in his chest again, Larry won't waste time before getting it checked out. "There is nothing wrong with getting a catheterization. If you feel a burn, check it out."

All his exercise, Larry thinks, will keep him healthier longer. "Think of Jim Fixx," he said. "He died of a heart attack. But by him exercising, the running, he lasted maybe five or ten years longer."

Now the exercise is more meaningful than ever. "I used to work out for the joy and the passion," Larry said. "Now I have to work out to keep me going. It's like medication."

Conclusion

Terry O'Neill was sitting at a bar in Pittsburgh, watching his favorite football team on the TV screen, when he was suddenly struck by a heart attack. Steelers' running back Jerome Bettis had just fumbled the ball late in a game on the two-yard line. Was there a connection? No one can say for sure, but we can play Monday morning quarterback and ask questions. The most important being, How aggressive had young Terry O'Neill been in looking after his own health? Had he fumbled the ball, too?

Jim Cantalupo, the sixty-year-old chief executive officer of McDonald's restaurants, collapsed and died of a heart attack while presiding over the corporation's annual convention in Orlando, Florida, in 2004.

Noted California labor leader Miguel Contreras died of a heart attack in 2005, at age fifty-two. And thirty-three-year-old Darryl Kile, a St. Louis Cardinal pitcher, died of a heart attack after complaining of chest pains in 2002.

ESPN commentator Michael Wilbon, then forty–nine, was in Phoenix in January 2008 to cover his twenty-first Super Bowl, but Wilbon didn't get to see the Patriots and Giants play. He suffered a heart attack and never made it to the game. But Wilbon survived, and got a scoop: While in the hospital to be treated for his heart attack, Wilbon learned that he was a diabetic and would need insulin injections for the rest of his "much healthier" life. His heart attack, like mine and so many others, proved to be a wakeup call, and a blessing.

I say it was grace that spared me when there are so many others who probably deserved this gift of life even more, but I appreciate the chance to put a few more days together. I get a complete and aggressive physical every year; my primary physician is a cardiologist who spares no effort when it comes to the heart health of his patients.

Heart attacks change people, and people who survive heart attacks can become change agents. Rev. James Love has made it part of his ministry to bring his heart-healthy lifestyle to his church members. Imagine how health-care costs would drop if every church followed his lead.

Anita Fox, Barbara Robinson, Mary Maguire, and Erin Peiffer have become advocates, not only for their own health but for the heart health of women in their communities.

For those people lucky enough to survive a heart attack, the key to a better existence is recognizing that this can be the beginning and not the end of life. We first learn to admit we have become sick, and then learn to accept our condition, which in most cases turns out to be only temporary.

Patience coupled with determination is needed before recovery can begin. We learn to trust others, starting with our doctors and nurses. We surrender to their care and advice.

We seek out and confide in others who have walked in our shoes or been confined to our beds.

Finally, we learn to cut ourselves, our families, and others some slack. We live in the now, taking each day one at a time. Tomorrow brings a totally new twenty-four hours. We have been given a reprieve from yesterday's mistakes. We will start the day anew. The Serenity Prayer usually works for me at the beginning of my morning: "God grant me the serenity to accept the things I cannot change, the courage to change the things I can, and the wisdom to know the difference."

American Heart Association Recommended Links

The site is organized around cardiovascular conditions and includes a glossary. http://www.heart.org.

HeartHub for Patients
http://www.hearthub.org/

Risk factors
http://www.americanheart.org/presenter.jhtml?identifier=4726

Calcification in the arteries
(See the section under EBCT—ultra-fast CT scanning)
http://www.americanheart.org/presenter.jhtml?identifier=4554

Oral health
http://www.americanheart.org/presenter.jhtml?identifier=3014399

Snoring/apnea
http://www.americanheart.org/presenter.jhtml?identifier=3058357

Heart and stroke encyclopedia http://www.americanheart.org/presenter.jhtml?identifier=10000056